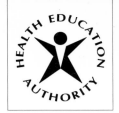

Effectiveness of video for health education: a review

J. Richard Eiser and Christine Eiser
Department of Psychology
University of Exeter

HEA Project Team
Jane Meyrick
Antony Morgan

HEA Project Team
Jane Meyrick   Research Project Manager
Antony Morgan   Head of Monitoring and Effectiveness Research

Special thanks are due to Cathy Herman and Angela Coulter for their commentaries and to Natalie Scaillet for assistance with the literature search.

In the same series:
Health promotion in older people for the prevention of coronary heart disease and stroke
Health promotion in childhood and young adolescence for the prevention of unintentional injuries

Forthcoming topics:
Young people and substance use
Young people and alcohol
Oral health
Healthy eating

For further information, tel. 0171 413 2624
To place an order, contact Marston Book Services, tel. 01235 465 565

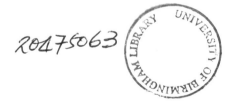

Designed by Edwin Belchamber
Typeset by Wayzgoose
Cover design by Raymond Loewy International Ltd
Printed in Great Britain

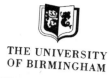

Contents

Structure of the report

The report begins with commentaries by Cathy Herman, Head of Health Promotion Information Services at the Health Education Authority and Mary Ryan also of the HEA, and Dr Angela Coulter, Director, King's Fund Development Centre about why the review was commissioned and a discussion of some of the issues raised by the authors' conclusions about the research evidence presented.

The report is then divided into three main sections: executive summary, main report and technical appendices.

The *executive summary* contains the main findings; summary of findings from each area reviewed; conclusions; future recommendations; and examples of best practice.

The *main report* begins by providing background details including the context and scope of the review; key questions addressed; theoretical basis of the studies; theoretical orientation of the reviews; and methodology. The report then presents all the studies reviewed, in detail, in Chapters 2 and 3, an evaluation of the social learning approach in Chapter 4 and a final summary and conclusion in Chapter 5.

The *technical appendices* present the authors' discussion of the main theoretical approaches. They also contain fuller details on the methodology used in the review; and a complete listing of all the studies in table form. The report concludes with full references to all the studies.

Commentary

Cathy Herman, Head of Health Promotion Information Services and Multimedia, HEA and Mary Ryan, Project Manager, Multimedia HEA

The Health Education Authority commissioned this review of effectiveness of video for health education to provide an overview of current knowledge concerning the effective production and use of this medium in the context of:

● an increase in the production and use of video for health education

● an increasing number of requests for information about the effectiveness of this medium

● the need to inform decision-making by both commissioners and providers of health education media

● the relatively high cost of producing video in comparison to other educational media

● to identify directions for future research and to contribute to an ongoing debate concerning evaluation and effectiveness of video.

The review confirms that video is a powerful tool for health educators. Visual messages can be used to engage and to emotionally involve the viewer and to personalise health education issues in a way which the written word cannot. Video can overcome difficulties with literacy. The visual nature of the medium is also preferred by some groups.

The review also contributes to the debates concerning the importance of the use of video within a well-planned intervention, the relevance of the context in which video is used and the need to actively involve the target audience in the planning and production of culturally appropriate media.

The review raises many issues and questions which will help to inform debate concerning the effectiveness of video and other educational media to support health promotion interventions. The review will be disseminated at a series of regional workshops where participants will have the opportunity to share learning and practice and to assist in identifying the next stages of this continuing work.

The rapid developments in interactive multimedia, of which video is a key component, are creating opportunities for the individual learner to define their own information and educational needs. However many of the issues raised by this review have equal relevance for the interactive media as for the more linear video programmes. Video will continue to be produced and used by health educators alongside the development of new media and we hope that this review will help to meet the need for information concerning effectiveness and the development and dissemination of best practice.

Commentary

Dr Angela Coulter, Director, King's Fund Development Centre

Those charged with the task of educating the public about the avoidance of health risks and the adoption of healthier lifestyles have an increasing array of tools at their disposal. Video offers great potential as a teaching aid because it avoids some of the limitations of written material, such as reliance on reasonable standards of literacy. A well-made video can engage the viewer much more directly than a leaflet and the combination of film, sound and graphics can be used creatively to impart new information, reinforce health education messages and demonstrate healthy behaviours and coping strategies. But video is expensive to produce, so it is important to find out whether, and in what circumstances, it is cost-effective.

This useful overview of the current state of knowledge of the effectiveness of video for health education contains some positive evidence that video has an important part to play. Some of the evaluations reviewed here demonstrate that video can be used to good effect as part of a carefully designed educational strategy. This is important because it shows that the effort of producing a video can be worthwhile, but we can also learn much from the failures and knowledge gaps documented in this critical review of the literature. The following issues are particularly important:

- Strategies intended to produce behaviour change must build on existing knowledge. There is a considerable body of research-based evidence on the factors that can promote or inhibit changes in behaviour and this has informed a number of coherent theories. Interventions using video are much more likely to succeed if they take account of what we already know.

- No teaching or decision aid is ever used in a vacuum, and video is no exception to this rule. Developers of videos must consider the context in which they will be used and the needs of the users. Video is usually more effective if it is part of a multi-component package, including supporting written material.

- The target audience and intended effects of the video should be clearly defined prior to production. The beliefs and attitudes of potential users should be researched and ideally they should be consulted at all stages of production.

● Videos are more likely to be effective if they actively engage people's attention. Interactive videos have obvious advantages, but it is often possible to introduce some interactivity into ordinary linear video.

● It is striking how many of the published 'evaluations' were so methodologically weak that we can learn little from them. This represents a huge waste of effort and resources. Far more attention should be devoted to the development of robust study designs, including randomised controlled trials and cost-effectiveness studies, so that future investment in video is informed by a sound body of evidence on what works, with which groups, in which contexts and at what cost.

Executive summary

Main findings

This review includes 175 studies involving the use of video in health education, using both health promotion and interventions within healthcare settings.
The review addressed the following key questions:

- *Is video effective in relation to short-/long-term knowledge gain, attitudinal and behavioural change?*

- Video *can* be effective in all these areas, but frequently fails for a variety of reasons.

- With respect to behaviour, many evaluations do not include measures of behaviour at all, and most of those which do, rely on self-reports without observational corroboration. Behavioural change is rarely produced simply through improved knowledge, but many interventions do not take other factors into consideration.

- With respect to knowledge and attitudes, several studies report modest improvements. However, many studies show little or no effect, presumably because of high levels of initial knowledge and positive attitudes ('ceiling effects').

- *Is video effective in relation to other media?*

- Few of the studies reviewed allow this question to be answered directly. Where video is used, it is often as part of a broader intervention programme, with little attempt made to identify the specific contribution of the video component.

- Where relevant comparisons can be drawn, results are mixed. Video does not automatically increase effectiveness, but may do so for specific issues and target groups.

- Multi-component interventions including video are generally more effective than video alone.

- *Is video effective as a medium for patient information?*

- Potentially, yes. However, this potential is still largely unfulfilled. More could be done, e.g. to use video to model self-care behaviours.

- Videos need to be presented in contexts where they will command patients' attention.

- Videos may be used to reassure patients before treatment, but may sometimes raise anxiety.

- *Can the use of modelling in video programmes bring about attitudinal or behavioural change?*

- Videos that use modelling are among the most effective in changing both attitudes and behaviour.

- Video is an ideal medium for interventions that encourage people to imitate specific behaviours.

- Social learning theory predicts that modelling is most likely to be effective when accompanied by opportunities for rehearsal and feedback.

Summary of findings from each area reviewed

AIDS and sexually transmitted diseases (STDs)

- Videos have been used successfully to model required behaviours among high-risk groups from more deprived backgrounds.

- It is unclear whether videos have any advantage over other techniques for raising awareness among more educated and less at-risk populations.

- Because of the number of different measures used, it is unclear whether video generally improves knowledge concerning AIDS and STDs.

Alcohol

- Theoretically-grounded interventions designed to teach specific relevant skills tend to be relatively successful.

- Interventions without a clear theoretical focus tend to be weaker, both methodologically and in terms of their findings.

Drugs

- Research in this area has tended to look for changes in attitudes and beliefs rather than actual behaviour.

- Video can be used to convey messages about the dangers of hard drugs and/or about the arguably arbitrary nature of the distinction between licit and illicit substances. These messages may not always seem consistent with each other, so the goals of any intervention should be clearly defined.

Smoking

- Interventions to train adolescents to resist social pressures to smoke have produced disappointing results.

- Interventions to motivate adults to quit, sometimes through vivid and personalised portrayal of health consequences, have had some success.

Nutrition

- Video can be a useful medium for nutritional education, but close attention needs to be paid to the information presented and the context of its presentation.

- Interventions that actively engage people's attention to such information while they are actually making decisions tend to have some impact.

- Interventions that depend on passive exposure to information generally have no effect.

Miscellaneous health promotion and prevention

- Modelling videos have been used successfully to promote blood donations among adolescents and to train younger children to avoid potential abductors.

- With adults, videos portraying health consequences have produced changes in intention, e.g. with respect to sun exposure and seat-belt use.

Preparation for surgery

- Positive effects have been found for video, although other forms of intervention also show success.

- Most work has involved patients with acute, rather than chronic, conditions.

Dentistry

- Interventions have generally failed to demonstrate reductions in patients' anxiety. This can probably be attributed to poor methodology and initial sample selection.

- The child's age and experience appear to interact with the intervention in determining the success of modelling videos.

Screening

- Results are encouraging for the use of videos to increase participation in cancer screening programmes, in particular among women from ethnic minorities.

- With advances in human genetics, counselling issues will need increasing attention.

Patient education

- Interventions in this area have mainly aimed to increase knowledge, but without using standard measures to evaluate effectiveness.

- It is unclear how gains in knowledge may translate to improved self-management.

- There could be considerable potential for videos that model practical self-management skills.

Parenting

- Suggestions that video could be useful for giving information to expectant and new parents, especially those in high-risk groups, need to be confirmed by sounder evaluations.

Conclusions

- Many published evaluations lack rigour, so findings need to be interpreted cautiously.

- Video can produce changes in attitudes and knowledge, but may not be generally more effective than other forms of intervention.

- Video can portray health consequences vividly and dramatically.

- Video tends to be more effective as part of an integrated programme than as a stand-alone intervention.

- Video can produce changes in behaviour through modelling, but effectiveness depends on a number of factors.

- Interventions without a clear theoretical framework almost always fail.

- Theoretically grounded interventions (particularly those based on social learning theory) tend to have greater success.

Future recommendations

- All interventions should specify the outcomes they seek to achieve, both immediately and in the longer term.

- A well-controlled design for evaluation (at least with respect to more easily measured outcome criteria) should be an integral part of the development of any intervention.

- Those developing video-based interventions should consider the context in which the videos are to be presented and how such presentations will be integrated with other available health education provision.

- Commissioners should consider the above conditions are met before funding the development or distribution of health education videos.

- There is considerable potential for development of video-based interventions for groups with special health needs. The active involvement of such groups or communities at all stages is essential.

- There is considerable potential for development of video-based interventions to model appropriate self-care behaviours among children and adults with chronic conditions.

- Interactive video has considerable potential for matching health education to individuals' need for information. Opportunities offered by new technology should be kept under review.

Examples of best practice

The following appear to us to be among the best examples of interventions that are both well planned and well evaluated. This selection includes studies on both children and adults, and is illustrative rather than exhaustive.

Children

We commend two studies, by the same research team, designed to teach young children how to get away from potential abductors (Carroll-Rowan and Miltenberger, 1994; Poche, Yoder and Miltenberger, 1988; 'Miscellaneous health promotion and prevention', 1, 4). These combine a modelling approach with feedback and behavioural rehearsal (as required by social learning theory). Positive aspects of the evaluations include a realistic test of acquired behavioural skills (despite ethical issues, which are sensitively handled) and a design permitting relevant comparisons (video *v.* training manual in 1; video with *v.* without rehearsal in 4; no treatment controls in both).

Adolescents

Few, if any, studies on adolescents in this review are clear examples of best practice. Although we have ourselves evaluated a major drug education programme ('Drugs', 2–6), this work suffers from a lack of integration between the programme development and evaluation phases. More commendable is a recent alcohol education study by Donaldson *et al.* (1995; see 'General references'), which distinguishes between correcting overestimations of the normativeness of drinking by peers, and training refusal skills. The critical interventions were not video-based and so the study is not part of this review. However, it is an example of a well-delivered programme submitted to careful evaluation.

Adults

We commend two studies evaluating sexual health interventions for ethnic minorities in American inner cities (Solomon and DeJong, 1988, 1989; 'AIDS', 16, 17). These are exemplary in terms of developing a programme with and for a particular community, a priority also demonstrated in more recent work from the same team (O'Donnell *et al.*, 1994; see 'General references'). They also include relevant behavioural measures – something that is not easily achieved in this area. McAvoy and Raza (1991; 'Screening', 5) confirmed the value of culturally sensitive video interventions in promoting uptake of cervical screening among Asian women. Banks *et al.* (1995; 'Screening', 1) demonstrated how a careful use of psychological theory in the design of persuasive messages can help promote participation in a breast-screening programme.

1. Introduction

Context of the review

This review was conducted over a four-month period from April 1995, following an invitation to tender from the HEA. This invitation stated that an extensive literature search had already been carried out for the period 1966–93, and we were asked to build upon this through updating the existing search up to January 1995, and allocating the studies 'along conventional and systematic lines of evaluation'. In practice, we found that the original literature search was incomplete in a number of respects. The main reason for this was that many articles appeared on computer searches only when we used keywords relating to specific health domains (e.g. 'nutrition') and did not appear under more general headings (e.g. 'health'). This implies that there may still be a number of potentially relevant articles we failed to find, relating to other specific health domains. Reflecting the methodology of our searches, therefore, the main body of this report will be organised around the literature relating to the use of video in separate health domains.

Scope of the review

Key questions

The key questions we were asked to consider in this review were as follows:

(a) Is video effective in relation to short-/long-term knowledge gain, attitudinal and behavioural change in relation to health education?

(b) Is video effective in relation to other media?

(c) Is video effective as a medium for patient information?

(d) Can the use of modelling in video programmes bring about attitudinal or behavioural change?

In addition, we were asked to comment on the extent to which the effectiveness of video might depend on other factors, such as the acceptability of the medium, cultural appropriateness, production style, context of use, and literacy level of the audience or user.

Are these questions answerable?

The reader should be warned at the outset that few of the studies to be reviewed are designed so as to provide direct answers to any of these questions (especially (a) and (b)). As will be described, the main focus in these studies has been on evaluating interventions that may include a more or less important element of video, but with the aim of assessing the impact of the intervention as a whole rather than the video element specifically.

Many interventions combine video with other educational techniques, such as group discussions led by peers or health professionals. Some of the most effective interventions (based on behavioural modelling) will also include a session in which participants rehearse specific responses. In such cases, it may be difficult, if not impossible, to identify the specific effect of video per se. On the other hand, in a broader context, this may not be the most significant issue. It may be of greater importance to consider theoretically the processes by which interventions of any kind can have a beneficial impact, and to consider practically how video can best contribute to this impact. This amounts to asking what one is attempting to achieve through any video intervention and how.

A few studies have attempted to present the same general information in video and non-video form, but it is difficult to know if the information presented is exactly the same across modalities, or if any conclusions drawn from such comparisons can be extrapolated to other kinds of messages. Others have presented different videos to different groups. In these the focus is on the kind of message rather than the medium through which it is presented. More generally, it must be recognised that 'video' is not a simple category. Over the time period covered by this review, both the technology itself and the manner of its use have changed dramatically. Likewise, no two videos will be exactly the same in terms of the ideas that have gone into their production, the theoretical assumptions about persuasion on which they are based, or the value positions which they espouse.

Theoretical bases of the studies

The studies reviewed are quite diverse with respect to the theoretical assumptions which guided the relevant interventions. These are described more fully in the technical report. The main approaches employed are, briefly:

(a) Informational approaches. Many studies aim simply to provide information, apparently assuming that improvement in knowledge (e.g. of health consequences) will lead to better behaviour.

(b) Attitude–intention–behaviour approaches. Other studies have been based on explicitly defined models about how different kinds of beliefs and evaluations contribute to a person's intention to perform a given behaviour. These beliefs may relate to the expected costs and benefits of the behaviour, social norms, perceived barriers to behavioural change and feelings of personal control. Best known among these models are the Health Belief Model, the Theory of Reasoned Action, and the Theory of Planned Behaviour.

(c) Social learning theory. This approach is the one associated with greatest success in the context of this review. This assumes that people will come to adopt behaviours for which they have been 'reinforced' (rewarded) and/or which they have witnessed being performed successfully by others. An advantage of this theory is that it specifies forms of intervention – especially those providing models for imitation – that are likely to be successful in producing behaviour change.

(d) Motivational approaches. A limited number of studies have attempted to differentiate individuals in terms of their receptiveness to health messages, as a function of either their personality or motivational readiness to change their behaviour.

Theoretical orientation of the review

Just as the studies can be differentiated according to whether or not they have been designed around a coherent theoretical framework, it is important for us to be explicit about our own theoretical premises adopted in this review. First, and most obviously, the perspective we adopt is a psychological one. Psychology is very largely concerned with how people assimilate information, form attitudes, and come to behave in particular ways. It therefore provides a conceptual and methodological framework within which to attempt to answer any questions concerning the impact of any intervention on knowledge, attitudes and behaviour.

The literature to be reviewed is also largely concerned with knowledge, attitudes and behaviour, but often not in a way which accords with current psychological thinking about the nature of these processes. In particular, we would question the seemingly widely-held presumption of a simple causal track from knowledge to attitude to intention to behaviour. When considering health behaviour, the appropriate model is rarely that of a deliberate decision-maker, weighing up the pros and cons of alternative options. Rather it is of a creature of habit, constrained by circumstances, who is predisposed through previous learning to act in particular ways, experience various hopes and fears, express particular opinions and attend to and recall particular kinds of information – all depending, to a great extent, on what comes easiest at the time. Both approaches can allow knowledge, attitudes and behaviour to be intercorrelated, but the meaning of these correlations will be interpreted very differently.

Clearly, the whole question of the effectiveness of health education interventions depends on which perspective one adopts. Presumably most interventions have as their ultimate aim the reduction of mortality or morbidity through behaviour change, but the strategies chosen to produce any such behaviour change are variable and often indirect. Crucially, if there is no 'royal road' to behaviour change from improved knowledge:

(a) Knowledge gain cannot be regarded as a simple predictor or surrogate measure of behaviour change.

(b) If an intervention is really aimed just at improving knowledge, it is critical to the definition of 'success' or 'effectiveness' to state whether improved knowledge is to be regarded as a desirable end in itself, or only worthwhile if it can be shown to lead ultimately to better health. This is in large part a judgement of value.

(c) If better health through behaviour change is indeed the desired end, one must either look specifically at how different kinds of information interact with prior attitudes and knowledge to influence behavioural choices or design interventions to have a direct impact on behaviour, conceivably bypassing knowledge and attitudes. In either case, this demands that interventions have a clear theoretical rationale. This will be one of the most important criteria we will employ in evaluating the studies described.

Methodology of the review

The studies to be reviewed were identified primarily from the PsychLIT and Medline databases. They have been grouped according to their relevance to eleven specific domains, within the two broad categories of (a) *health promotion and prevention* and (b) *healthcare settings*.

The diversity of the studies identified required a more flexible approach than that suited to more conventional clinical reviews. The latter tend, very properly, to exclude from consideration studies that fail to incorporate common outcome measures or to meet basic standards of experimental design and control (such as those employed in randomised clinical trials of a new medical procedure). This kind of approach is appropriate where one is reviewing studies that all employ similar procedures to answer the same, or similar, questions. However, it would have been unworkable in the present context because of the theoretical and methodological diversity of the studies identified.

The main obstacle is that not all interventions share a common aim. Whereas some seek to modify specific health-related behaviours, others merely aim to raise awareness of broader health issues. Hence, no single set of outcome measures can be used to decide if an intervention has 'worked'. Even so, it is important to decide whether the outcome measures employed in a given study are appropriate for the aims of the intervention, so particular attention will be given to this in the review.

Another problem is that much of the evidence relates to the effectiveness of interventions of which video is a *part*, but do not attempt to identify how much of any effect is attributable to video per se, as distinct from other parts of the intervention. Hence, we could not restrict our review to studies employing simple 'video intervention' *v.* 'no video control'. Again, our review will attempt to indicate what inferences can or cannot be drawn from specific studies, in view of the design employed.

Finally, it is unfortunately the case that many of the published studies lack rigour and so cannot be regarded as offering dependable conclusions. These would obviously have been excluded from a conventional clinical review. However, we believed it was more instructive to include them, but to comment on their shortcomings. In this way, we hope our review may not simply provide a summary of previous findings, but offer some suggestions for future evaluation research.

Referencing of studies

Individual studies included in the review will be referenced numerically rather than by authors' names. The numerical codes apply within each specific domain (e.g. 'Smoking'; 'Alcohol') separately, and are used in the tables in Appendix C and for the list of references at the end of the report. Literature reviews specific to particular domains are referenced by authors' names and are listed at the end of the references for the relevant domain. More general articles, e.g. theoretical or methodological papers, or studies of relevance to our discussion but not meeting the inclusion criteria of this review, are referenced by authors' names and listed under 'General references' at the end of the report.

2. Review of studies on the use of video in health promotion and prevention

Introduction

All the studies reviewed in this chapter relate to contexts where people's behaviour directly influences their health status and vulnerability to illness or injury. One might expect that behavioural change would therefore be an immediate and consistent aim of the interventions reported. In fact this is not always the case. Sometimes this is because of the difficulty of establishing that behavioural change has become established within the time-frame available for evaluation (as in some of the studies on smoking and alcohol use) and sometimes because the behaviours in question are performed privately (safer sex practices, illicit drug use and, to some extent, eating habits). Another, possibly more influential, reason is that many interventions have adopted a more indirect approach. At its best, this may be interpreted as an attempt not simply to combat the problematic behaviours, but their presumed underlying causes in the knowledge, attitudes, and general self-confidence and social skills of the individuals. This presumption of an underlying causal process has guided a number of interventions, particularly those adopting a 'life-skills' approach to the prevention of smoking and drug-abuse in young people. The evaluations are therefore often at least as much a test of the underlying approach as of the effectiveness of the medium.

The reader will discern considerable differences between the styles of interventions aimed at young people on the one hand, and adults on the other. Most of the former are based on some version of a social learning approach, either with a broad emphasis on life-skills or a narrower focus on 'inoculation' against persuasion and the training of specific resistance strategies. Despite this, there is variation between the areas in how effectively these ideas have been put into practice. Adolescent smoking prevention programmes appear to be some of the most disappointing, both in the sensitivity with which they have been developed and, in some cases, in the soundness of the evaluations.

As in many other areas, we need to ask whether the fault lies more with the underlying theory or the manner in which it has been applied.

Recently, Donaldson *et al.* (1995) evaluated an alcohol education programme not based on video. They concluded that resistance-skills training may delay onset of alcohol use by adolescents, but only if students have also received 'normative education' to correct their tendency to overestimate the incidence and social acceptability of alcohol use among their peers.

The studies on adults are more of a mixed bag. Included are a number of frankly very poor reports, employing inadequate samples and/or designs to evaluate interventions that seem to do little more than offer a mixture of health facts and exhortations, without any clear theoretical rationale. However, there are also a number of excellent interventions, where the required changes in behaviour are tightly specified and imaginatively communicated. More attitudinally-based interventions also report some success, perhaps because their producers (often, broadcasters) have been less inhibited in their inclusion of more shocking material. Again there are differences between areas, but perhaps more important are those between studies performed on undergraduate students, who often may be relatively unconcerned with the health issue in question, and those involving general public samples (e.g. employees in workplace studies) and high-risk groups for whom the decisions really matter.

AIDS and STDs

We identified 27 eligible studies on AIDS and sexually transmitted diseases (STDs), of which 25 were American, 1 was from Australia and 1 from India. Granted the global nature of the AIDS epidemic, this distribution is bizarre. Doubtless this does not reflect the amount of effort being devoted to intervention programmes (with and without video) in many other countries. However, there is a possibility that many such programmes are not being systematically evaluated. Despite this national bias, this set of studies is relatively diverse. Six of the studies (1–6) involve adolescents and/or families, eleven (7–17) use 'high-risk' or patient groups, and ten (18–27) use undergraduate students.

The main emphasis is on teaching safer sex practices, especially condom use. Examples of behavioural measures that go beyond self-report are being tested for HIV (9), obtaining condoms (3, 9, 17, 22), and clinic re-attendance (16). While interventions in this field benefit from being able to state clear behavioural recommendations, researchers are divided in terms of their emphasis on behavioural or attitude change, with less than half of the evaluations testing for effects on self-reported and/or observed behaviour. This reticence is reflected in previous discussions. In a review of eight previous studies, Healton and Messeri (1993) concluded that videos may be effective in changing attitudes and knowledge, but that they tended to have little impact on behaviour.

Likewise, Winett and Anderson (1994), while arguing for the importance of training families and adolescents in problem-solving skills, warn against over-reliance on measures of intention as surrogate measures of behaviour among younger respondents.

Effectiveness is assessed against a variety of comparison conditions, often other videos of different style and content. These can include factual videos about AIDS as opposed to those modelling safer practices. The prize for curiosity must go to one study (22) which compared videos demonstrating condom use with a 'control' film about radio-controlled aeroplanes! Two of the strongest studies (16, 17) use a simple no-intervention control in an after-only design. The studies divide almost equally between those adopting an atheoretical 'informational' approach and those based on an identifiable rationale (mainly social learning, but also other models of decision-making and attitude change).

The six studies on *adolescents* include two by the same research group (5, 6) using a social learning/modelling approach to improve AIDS-related knowledge and problem-solving skills among adolescents and their families. The results are encouraging for the use of video interventions on sensitive topics within a family setting, as opposed to more typical classroom-based programmes from which other family members are clearly excluded.

A third study is based on a combination of the theory of reasoned action and social learning, but merely tests for acceptability (1). A fourth reports negative findings for an informational intervention aimed at adolescents at a residential centre (4). This leaves a pair of studies (2, 3) both by the same authors which are some of the best based on an informational approach. The first also tested for behaviour (exchanging coupons for condoms), and although no overall advantage for the video programme was found, within this intervention group those who had used condoms before were more likely to redeem the coupons. The second study compared peer-led and adult-led approaches; both conditions showed an advantage over controls but did not differ from each other.

Considered as a group, the studies on *'high-risk'* groups provide good evidence for the effectiveness of video programmes, but only when these are based on a clear theoretical perspective, particularly social learning/modelling. A study of unmarried women of whom some were at high risk (10) showed increases in self-efficacy and preventive behaviours such as condom purchases, particularly when modelling was reinforced by cognitive rehearsal. In an excellent study (16) involving 1153 STD clinic outpatients with gonorrhea from a predominantly black inner-city sample, a modelling intervention greatly improved re-attendance at the clinic for 'test of cure' examination. The rationale for this study incorporates both social learning and the health belief model.

A further study by the same authors (17) with a similar sample found an effect on redeeming coupons for free condoms. The one Australian study (14), which applied a social learning approach in an intervention targeted at homosexual men, found no differences between the impact of video and other programmes, but this appears to be due to a ceiling effect, with most of the sample having very positive attitudes to safe sex beforehand.

Interventions less explicitly based on this perspective yield less success in terms of behavioural change. Negative findings are reported by most interventions aimed at high-risk groups using an 'informational' approach (7, 8, 12). One study reporting positive behavioural change among high-risk Afro-American women (9) has been classified as 'informational', in that its theoretical rationale is less clearly stated, but it appears much closer to studies using a decision-making approach than the others in this category. Another study without a clearly stated theoretical perspective (13), but implicitly adopting a coping approach, reports successful reduction of anxiety relating to HIV testing.

Possibly the most difficult study in this set to evaluate is the one targeted at Delhi prostitutes (15). This reports a gain in awareness of AIDS and self-reported condom use over a two-year period – and a lack of increase in a (suspiciously low) rate of HIV – as a consequence of an ambitious programme involving video and peer communicators. This appears to have many of the hallmarks of a sensitively planned programme with community involvement. However, the absence of a control group is especially unfortunate. The design does not exclude the possibility that these changes would have occurred historically over this period, irrespective of any intervention, or reassure the reader that the findings do not partly reflect self-selection into the sample by those more concerned to practise safer sex.

The studies on *undergraduates and adults* show a mixture of positive effects, in terms of knowledge increase and more favourable attitudes towards condoms. The involvement of such subjects with the issue seems much less than that of the higher-risk groups. Of the three studies considering attitudes towards AIDS victims, one (25) uses employees rather than students, with the issue being attitudes towards an infected co-worker. Some increase in sympathy was reported, but not for subjects with antihomosexual attitudes. Of the two using student subjects, one also showed some increase in sympathy (24) but the other (18) suggested messages emphasising the avoidability of HIV infection may lead to a less tolerant and blaming attitude.

All in all, these studies are encouraging for the prospects of using videos to model required behaviours among high-risk groups from more deprived backgrounds. It is less clear that videos have any advantage over other techniques for raising awareness among more educated and less at-risk populations. Conclusions regarding the impact of video on knowledge concerning AIDS and STDs are made even more difficult because of the number of different measures in use.

Alcohol

We identified 17 eligible articles concerned with alcohol use, including 12 from the USA, 3 from the UK, and 1 each from Australia and Canada. These are of variable quality. Five were aimed at teenagers, six at patients with drinking problems, and six at other adult groups.

Of those using *adolescents*, two by Duryea (3, 4) are based on McGuire's Inoculation Theory and employ the powerful Solomon 4-group design. The interventions here consist of video plus supportive sessions and role-play, with the main aim of training pupils to refute arguments that play down the dangers of drink-driving (4 is a replication of 3). Both report positive effects on ability to refute arguments, and on self-reported behaviour (drinking and riding with a drink-driver). A third (1) provides experimental evidence of the value, for attitude change, of matching the sex of a communicator with that of the target. The remaining two studies are weak. One (2) is a small-scale report of an atheoretical intervention in two classes of a single school. The other (5), again atheoretical, suggests some change in attitude against drink-driving and drinking when pregnant but no statistical tests were apparently performed!

The six on *patients* with drinking problems include four (7, 8, 9, 10) that employ a social learning/behavioural modelling approach to train patients to adopt and/or recognise desired behaviours. The first (7) finds improvements on specific observed behavioural indices, such as drinking speed, for a video modelling controlled drinking, although it was even more effective to play back to patients a video-recording of their own drinking behaviour. Two (8, 9) successfully use a modelling approach to get detoxification patients to seek further treatment. A fourth (10) also successfully employs a social learning/modelling approach to teach two inmates of Rampton Hospital with learning disabilities and drinking problems to identify strategies for reduced drinking. The other two studies (6, 11) test for knowledge gain rather than behaviour change, but find no advantage for video.

The remaining studies on *college students* and other *adults* form a more diverse set. One (16) adopts a social learning approach to train a small sample of students described as 'heavy social drinkers' to moderate their consumption. This reports some success for an intervention package involving a modelling video and practice training, but not for another video that merely explained the rationale for a moderate drinking style.

This is therefore quite similar to studies 7–10. The remainder all adopt an informational approach. The impact of video interventions is confined to improvement in knowledge, but two studies (12, 17) fail to achieve even this. Perhaps the most disappointing findings come from a large British study of 2100 pregnant women (17), where a video designed to point out the risks of drinking when pregnant aroused little interest and had no effect on knowledge and behaviour compared with a leaflet. Another large-scale British study (15) reports the results of a survey of audience reactions to a television-based campaign in Scotland. Viewers of the campaign scored higher on knowledge than non-viewers, as well as differing in various demographic characteristics. However, the authors conclude that there was no evidence of an increase in knowledge about alcoholism or reduction of alcohol consumption among the Scottish population as a whole during the period of the campaign.

Although quite diverse, this set of studies implies that theoretically grounded interventions designed to teach specific relevant skills, either argumentative (3, 4) or behavioural (7–10, 16), tend to be relatively successful in achieving their aims. Those that lack a clear theoretical focus are less impressive, both in terms of their findings and, in some cases, in the methodology applied in their evaluation.

Drugs

There are surprisingly few studies specifically evaluating the use of video in drug education (although marijuana use is sometimes considered along with tobacco; see 'Smoking' 2, 15). Only 8 eligible studies were identified, of which we ourselves were the authors of 5. Hence, the typical predominance of American work is not found in this domain. All the studies employ secondary or high school samples (one uses teachers) and all but one use some version of a social learning/life-skills approach. The emphasis is on primary prevention rather than on changing the behaviour of those who are already habitual users of drugs. Direct evidence of effects on behaviour is lacking. Only one study (1) obtained self-reports of previous use of illicit drugs (marijuana), using this as a predictor of intentions and reactions to the message. Otherwise behavioural self-reports concerned (under-age) use of tobacco and alcohol (3, 4) and use of refusal skills (6), none of which was consistently affected by the interventions.

There is stronger evidence for the influence of video-based interventions on attitudes and knowledge. However, the form and direction of this influence reflects the content of the videos. The most relevant studies on this point (2–6) are those evaluating the DHSS drug education package *Double Take* offered free to all secondary schools in England and Wales during 1986. This included two videos, very different in style and emphasis. One (the most popular with teachers and students) was a specially scripted episode of the television drama series *Minder*. This featured a teenage boy, some of whose acquaintances start taking heroin. While resistance to social pressure is a dominant theme, so also is the fact that drugs such as heroin are addictive and potentially lethal. The second video, called *Thinking Twice*, mainly consists of discussions and factual presentations by young actors. Again, social pressures are discussed, but the message is more 'Here are some things you should know so you can decide for yourselves'. Among the facts presented are those which point out how the term 'drug' could apply to many licit substances (including caffeine). The evidence, most directly from experimental comparison (5), is that these two videos had different, and sometimes opposite effects. The *Minder* video was very effective in impressing on young people the dangers of illicit drug use, while alerting them to the importance of situational pressures. *Thinking Twice*, on the other hand, led students to regard licit substances as more dangerous, but illicit drugs as somewhat less so. Girls were more sympathetic to the idea of dealing with drug use in the context of general personal development.

An important issue raised by research in this area is that of which specific attitudes and beliefs one is seeking to change. The meaning of 'drug use' depends on which substances are labelled as drugs. It is possible to use video to convey messages about the dangers of hard drugs and about the arguably arbitrary nature of the distinction between licit and illicit substances. However, there is a risk that these aspects of drug education can act against each other, at least when outcome is measured in terms of global evaluations. The use of video as a medium, therefore, would seem to be less critical than the content of the message.

Smoking

We identified 28 eligible studies concerning smoking (or more precisely, 26 plus 2 on smokeless tobacco use). Of these, 22 were from the USA, 5 from the UK and 1 from Germany. Fifteen (1–15) were concerned with adolescents, with the aim of preventing uptake. The remainder (16–28) used adults, with the main aim of persuading smokers to quit.

With these aims in mind, one might expect all the studies to include a measure of behaviour, at least at the level of self-report. Biochemical validation of smoking self-reports (e.g. exhaled CO, salivary thiocyanate) is feasible, but the time and expense of collecting and analysing such data is far from trivial, and one should not be too censorious when such procedures are omitted. (Generally speaking, self-reports of smoking consumption, when checked against such validation measures, tend to be reasonably honest.) However, it is less easy to establish an outcome of change in smoking *behaviour* as an effect of an intervention. One reason may be that smoking is partly under the control of many systems of reinforcement, including pharmalogical, which an educational intervention by itself could not be fairly expected to overcome. An even more direct reason is that evidence of change takes time to appear. As far as behaviour change is concerned, an immediate post-test is not enough. In studies of smoking cessation, it is likely to take weeks or even months to establish whether smokers have been persuaded to quit or reduce their consumption. In studies of prevention, programmes may aim to teach cognitive and personal skills to 12-year-olds to deter them from becoming smokers at any time over the next four to five years. Because of this, a number of studies have concentrated on more proximal variables, such as attitudes and intention. Most, however, have attempted to include at least self-reports of behaviour and to measure effectiveness over a more extended period.

The fifteen studies relevant to *adolescent smoking prevention* include some of the most ambitious in this review. At first sight, most of the studies have the features of well planned and evaluated research. Large samples are the norm. A theoretical rationale can be readily identified, and throughout this is some variant of a social learning approach, with emphases on life-skills modelling and 'inoculation' against pro-smoking messages. Although the health risks of smoking are considered, these are not the main focus of communication, since there is a presumption that these are already known. Important exceptions are the two studies on smokeless tobacco use (4, 14), where an explicit aim is to impress on adolescents the riskiness of this activity. Elsewhere, the dominant notion is that intervention should teach adolescents to resist social pressures to smoke. These pressures are thought to include peer-group influence, parental and other adult models and commercial advertising.

The first major study to adopt this approach was that by Evans *et al.*, 1981 (3). This claimed significant success in inhibiting smoking onset among teenagers over a three-year period. These claims encouraged the development of many similar programmes in the USA and other countries, including the UK. However, closer inspection of the analyses reported in this study reveals that these are seriously flawed. Basically, the evaluation is set up as though it is a longitudinal study with several repeated measures, with different junior high schools randomly allocated to receive different interventions. However, it is impossible to track the progress of any individual pupils over the three years. The authors therefore fall back on so-called 'cross-sectional' comparisons between school groups at different times. The trouble with this, though, is that the composition of the groups themselves appears very unstable, with movement between, into and away from, the schools used. It is impossible to distinguish the results for those pupils who remained in the cohort throughout, or to determine if attrition was non-randomly associated with smoking status (e.g. if would-be smokers were more likely to drop out from the intervention groups).

However, even if we set aside the results of this study, the remainder in this set provide little positive evidence for a specific impact of video-based interventions. Another influential life-skills approach to smoking and use of other drugs (2) reports significant success rates for the programme as a whole (in New York high schools). However, video was used only to train the teachers who administered this programme, and showed no advantage in this regard over other forms of training. One study (7) used an interactive video to teach specific 'refusal skills' (how to say no to an offer of a cigarette) and found a positive effect on assessment of these skills in a standardised role-play; however, this involved a small sample and the researchers conducting the assessment may not have been blind to the experimental condition of the subjects. Positive results on validated change in smoking behaviour come from another small-scale study (12). A larger study (15) compared effects on self-reported smoking of three conditions: video plus peer-led discussion, video only, and a no-intervention control. The first condition showed an inhibition of onset of smoking over the school year compared with the other two conditions (with some generalisation to alcohol and marijuana). However, video without peer-led discussion showed no advantage over the control group. Even more negative findings come from one study (6) in which video was used as a control group against which to evaluate a programme built around structured discussions of different risk factors. This programme was significantly better than video in inhibiting young adolescents' progress from their first to their second cigarette.

This leaves evaluations of impact on attitudes and knowledge, and once again the evidence is somewhat discouraging, with only three studies other than those already cited reporting positive effects. One of these (13) is essentially an exploration of the feasibility of family-based interventions, and focuses on attitudes of teenagers and parents to parental involvement in smoking prevention. The remaining two (4, 14) both concern the issue of smokeless tobacco use, where, one might surmise, the health risks are generally less recognised and acknowledged. The second of these also includes an interesting manipulation of styles of presentation of risk information.

Turning to the 13 studies on *adult smoking*, one finds an emphasis on devising approaches to encourage smokers to quit. There are also a few smaller-scale experiments which are not strictly interventions, but which provide some evidence about how individuals may interpret fear-arousing messages about smoking risks. Two studies (17, 26) report successful behavioural change with biochemical validation as a consequence of interventions including video. One (17) compares an aversive (rapid smoking) therapy with a 'health motivation' intervention including a minor element of video. The latter intervention was more successful than the former, but there was no 'no-treatment' control group. Another (26) found encouraging results on cessation for a brief intervention aimed at general hospital inpatients. This included a video and a bedside counselling session. A study on primary care patients (20) reports positive behavioural effects, but the criterion here is attendance at a smoking cessation programme rather than actual success at cessation. These last two studies are based on the notions of motivational readiness to change (Prochaska and DiClemente, 1983).

Three more studies (19, 25, 27) report positive effects on self-reported behaviour. One (19) uses a self-selected sample with no control group, so the results are of little value. The other two both investigate the effects of videos with *fear-arousing messages*. One of these (25) is a small-scale experiment (from Germany) more concerned with people's interpretations of their own emotional reactions, but still finds greater change in self-reported smoking and intentions under conditions where subjects felt more frightened by a 40-minute television film about smoking. A British television film (*Dying for a Fag*) is also the intervention in the second of these articles (27), which reports two studies in which the comparison conditions involve showing a television film about either alcohol abuse or seat belts. Smokers who saw the anti-smoking film reported stronger intentions to quit and were more likely to have tried to stop or cut down by the time of follow-up. The analyses focus on the impact of the film on intervening variables such as fear and other health beliefs. However, a later paper from the same research group (18) summarising a series of studies on smoking interventions in workplace settings found little or no positive impact for (minimal) video-based interventions, which were significantly less effective than treatment with nicotine gum. Two further studies (both British) pursue the fear-arousal theme: one (28) is a tiny study of female hospital staff, suggesting that smokers showed greater anxiety and intention to quit after viewing the same television film used in study 27. The second (16) is a report of audience reactions to another anti-smoking television documentary (*Smokers' Luck*). Although the report implies an impact on attitudes and intention, the lack of a comparison with non-viewers means that this cannot be assessed. More informative is the finding that the sample of viewers included fewer heavy smokers than would be expected by chance, implying self-selection against exposure to such messages. No other studies report any advantage for video-based interventions.

Despite the obvious importance of smoking for many areas of health, and the effort that has consequently gone into devising anti-smoking interventions, this group of evaluation studies makes somewhat depressing reading.

With respect to adolescents, programmes built around notions of social learning and life-skills training can have some positive impacts (2), but it is less certain how cost-effective these generally are in terms of staff and curriculum time. There is little evidence that video is needed for these programmes to be effective. Similar reservations are expressed in a review by Flay (1985) evaluating earlier 'resisting social pressures' interventions. Concluding that 'the social influences approach to smoking prevention can be effective on some adolescents some of the time' (p. 93), he calls for, among other things, more attention to intervening psychological processes, more consideration of how interventions may be delivered other than by professional researchers, and a following-through of refinements to such programmes, such as role-playing and explicit rehearsal of behavioural skills.

On the other hand, the fault may sometimes lie less with the medium and presentation than with the content of the message. Many researchers seem to have taken it for granted that the main reason young people start to smoke is because they lack the skills to resist social pressures. Merely showing that young smokers have smoking friends does not establish the presence of coercive influence: it may simply reflect friendship choice based on similarity (see Eiser *et al.*, 1991). If this assumption of social pressures is incorrect, even the most cleverly-devised programme to teach resistance skills will have little impact on smoking.

Before deciding to use video to model certain skills, one needs to be sure that these skills are the ones required for behavioural change. Whereas many areas of health education suffer from a lack of theoretical direction, here the problem seems to be more one of a premature theoretical commitment which has steered researchers away from other interpretations.

Along with commitment to the idea of resisting social pressures, another piece of received wisdom is that smokers 'already know' the risks that they are running. Against this, some of the more positive findings from this set of studies are those dealing with the less familiar risks of smoke-less tobacco, and also those that imply that fear-arousal can have a direct effect on attitudes and intentions.

There is an important difference between 'knowing' about risks and actually considering them. Something the video medium can do very effectively is to portray health consequences in more memorable and personally relevant ways, although there is always a possibility that some people will avoid messages that they dislike. It is noteworthy that examples of this 'harder' use of video to communicate health messages come from broadcasters rather than health educators.

Nutrition

Ten studies were identified concerned with nutrition and directed at the general population. (There are additional articles concerned with the provision of more specific dietary advice to patients with different diseases, which are described in the relevant 'Patient Education' sections.) All 10 studies are from the USA. The aim tends to be to encourage awareness and adoption of low-fat high-fibre diets, primarily so as to reduce the risk of cardiovascular disease, although one intervention (1) focuses on reduction of cancer risk.

Only two of the articles deal with *children*. One (5) describes two interventions directed at 13- to 14-year-old girls and concentrates on attitudes to weight control and avoidance of bulimia. Dietary intentions improved relative to controls following a video plus discussion session. The second (7) used a sophisticated version of an informational approach to evaluate the responses of 5- to 6-year-olds to excerpts from television programmes and advertisements for nutritious foods. Improvement in nutritional knowledge, attitudes and observed behaviour (food choice) was found for both intervention and control groups, with a non-significant advantage for the former. However, the statistical treatment of the data is unusually conservative and might disguise a real effect.

Two studies (3, 4) evaluate the effects of dietary advice provided to *adults* identified through workplace cholesterol screening as being at higher cardiovascular risk. Of these, the first is the more theoretically based (on the Health Belief Model), and the more successful in producing improvements in knowledge, attitudes and behaviour, especially among participants with lower educational levels. A third (6) deals with men with high cholesterol already attending a clinic. This showed modest improvements in self-reported breakfast diet as a consequence of viewing a video with or without discussion.

The five remaining studies (1, 2, 8, 9, 10) are based in supermarkets and consider the impact of a variety of video techniques on nutritional attitudes and choice. The first two involved playing short films and public service announcements about better nutrition on video screens while shoppers made their purchases. While these presentations were rated as acceptable, they attracted little attention and seemed to have essentially no effect. Far more successful are the last three studies, all by the same authors, based on a social learning approach. These employed *interactive video* interventions, in which customers received advice and feedback with respect to their food purchases, whereas controls merely used the system to record their purchases. Increased purchasing of high-fibre foods was found as a result of the interventions.

Taken as a whole, these suggest that video can be a useful medium for nutritional education, but that close attention needs to be paid to the information presented and the context of its presentation. Interventions that actively engage people's attention to such information while they are actually making decisions tend to have some impact. Those that depend on passive exposure to information generally do not.

Miscellaneous health promotion and prevention

Twelve studies were grouped within this category, 6 on children and adolescents and 6 on adults. There were 6 studies from the USA, 2 from the UK, 2 from Canada, 1 from Australia and 1 from Surinam.

Those on *younger* samples form an interesting set. Two studies (1, 4) from the same research team employed a modelling/social learning approach to teach young children (4–7 years) necessary verbal and avoidance behaviours to repel a *potential abductor*. These assessed effectiveness by having a researcher actually approach the children as though to abduct them and observe their responses. In both studies, although a video showing the required behaviours led to safer responses than a control condition, far better results were obtained when the video presentation was combined with rehearsal of the required behaviours. These studies present strong evidence for the effectiveness of a full application of the precepts of social learning theory. The theme of protection from assault continues in a less theoretically-based, and less conclusive, study on 9- to 13-year-olds (6), in which children were encouraged to think about their feelings in response to different kinds of approaches by adults.

Another study using a social learning approach describes a large-scale programme to promote blood donation (5). The video contained specific behavioural instructions on how to participate in the blood drive, along with modelling to increase positive attitudes and reduce anxieties. Elements of a modelling approach are also discernible in a description of a programme to combat *infection* among elementary and junior high-school students in rural Surinam (2), many of whom had no previous experience of television. Unfortunately, no quantitative analysis is reported, but quotations from interviews with children provide qualitative indications that the video was both acceptable and instructive, although it proved difficult to communicate the whole range of ways in which infection could spread. This leaves a well-planned informational intervention to improve adolescents' knowledge about *blood pressure* (3). This showed an advantage of video over a leaflet when knowledge was assessed at one week, though not at follow-up.

Among the studies on *adult* samples, three evaluate video interventions to promote protection against skin cancer from *sun exposure*. An Australian study (7), based on the Health Belief Model, presented undergraduates with either a factual or emotional video about the risks of skin cancer, while a control group saw a film about heart disease. Both relevant videos improved intentions for sun protection relative to controls. Persistence of this effect was greater in response to the emotional video, although the factual video produced greater gains in knowledge. An American study (9) found that a video portraying a young woman needing treatment for skin lesions succeeded in changing students' expressed stereotypes concerning the attractiveness of a suntan, and lessened their optimism regarding their own personal level of risk. Both these studies, however, were conducted in university settings and extrapolation to actual behaviour, and to the general population, deserves further consideration. However, the one general population study on this issue (10) is weak. The only outcome measure is whether beachgoers attended a video presentation, as opposed to accepting other forms of intervention (e.g. free samples of skin care products). Since they had to leave the beach to see the video, it is unsurprising that few agreed to participate!

Of the three remaining studies, one is an evaluation of six health promotion videos produced for US Navy personnel (8). These were presented with and without discussion sessions. Increases in knowledge were found only for a video on back injuries, with no difference depending on whether there was a discussion. The topics of the other (ineffective) videos were tobacco, fitness, stress, drugs and alcohol, and nutrition. The impact of the interventions was restricted to improvements in knowledge. Two (11, 12) assess the impact of a fear-arousing film about road accidents on intentions to wear seat-belts. Like other papers by the same authors concerning smoking ('Smoking' 18, 27), these imply that fear-arousal can be an important motivator of certain forms of behaviour change, and that the effects of such communications can be tracked through relevant cognitive intervening variables, such as risk beliefs.

3. Review of studies on use of video in healthcare settings

Introduction

Patients need information. Not only is there a moral duty for physicians to provide information, but increasingly this is acknowledged also to be a legal obligation. Potentially videos offer the opportunity to provide information systematically, to be efficient with regard to the use of professional time, and to provide a back-up to more conventional forms of doctor–patient communication. Apart from providing general information, videos have enormous potential in teaching individual skills including, for example, teaching patients with diabetes how to self-inject insulin, or those with asthma the correct use of an inhaler.

Given the extent to which videos could be used in healthcare settings, it is disappointing to find so few genuine evaluations. We are aware of a large number of videos which have been produced by hospitals and charities concerned with preparing patients for hospital admission generally, or related to specific diseases. Regrettably, very few of these have been formally evaluated.

A number of previous reviews were identified. All criticise the methodologies in practice, but point to the value of video in healthcare settings generally. Our review, while including much more recent material points nevertheless to related conclusions.

Preparation for surgery

We identified 20 articles concerned with preparing patients for surgery or medical investigations; 12 focused on children and the remainder on adults. All the work with children was conducted in the USA; all but two of the adult studies were also (one article was Australian and one from Germany).

The main goals were to (a) reduce anxiety and fear prior to surgery or intervention, as measured by self-report or inferred from physiological indicators; and (b) encourage appropriate and cooperative behaviour during procedures (especially among young children).

We found a number of well-designed studies in this area; the majority of which were grounded in firm theoretical ideas. These largely include social learning theory (11), information (6) and coping (1), cognitive development (1) and behaviour modification (1).

Especially in work with *children*, there is a heavy emphasis on measuring fear or anxiety (9) and observer ratings of behaviour (11). There is less emphasis on physiological measures and symptoms (1) or knowledge (2). This is in contrast to *adult* work, where there is much less emphasis on observer-rated behaviour (3), though interest in self-rated mood or anxiety (8) and knowledge (5) is higher.

In comparison with other interventions, there is much to suggest that videos can be used successfully in this area. Positive effects were reported on physiological symptoms (1), observer-rated behaviours (10), self-rated mood or anxiety (10), and knowledge (2).

Where more detailed comparisons have been conducted between videos and more than one form of intervention, videos have been reported to be better than a nurse intervention but poorer than a class-based package (9), and a previsit to the hospital better than video in reducing maternal anxiety (12).

Previous reviews have generally been favourable concerning the value of videos, especially those based on social learning principles (Melamed, 1977; Saille *et al.*, 1988). The meta-analysis reported by Saille *et al.* (1988) is worthy of special consideration. They conducted a meta-analysis of studies published between 1953 and 1985 concerned with preparation of children for medical and surgical procedures. They concluded that almost any type of intervention could be regarded as successful. However, modelling interventions (which were the most frequent), were found to be less successful than other methods. (However, this may be an artifact of the way in which meta-analyses are conducted. The suggestion that modelling procedures were less successful was based on a larger number of studies compared with other methods and therefore the conclusion that other methods are superior may be based on the results of just one study.)

As with other reviews, we conclude that there is substantial evidence that preparation for hospitalisation and surgery is beneficial for children and adults, and that there is little systematic evidence to suggest that any single preparatory method is superior. To a large extent, we support the conclusions made by others that hospitals can choose between different forms of preparation depending on their resources, budget and purpose.

This conclusion should be tempered by some reservations about the way previous studies have been conducted and particularly the inadequacies of outcome measures typically used. The literature is difficult to interpret because there are differences between studies in the samples investigated. There remains little work on patients with chronic or severe conditions and much more on those with acute problems. The question of the most appropriate timing of interventions remains unclear and is almost certainly confounded by the child's age. Finally, it would be irresponsible not to mention that there is evidence that preparation can have negative effects especially for some subgroups. These include children with previous hospital experience (see Faust and Melamed, 1984).

Increasingly it is acknowledged that at least as far as children are concerned, parental attitude and behaviour are critical. The development of a new generation of videos may well benefit from recent work, documenting more systematically how parents attempt to answer children's questions, and their use of distraction and coping techniques which encourage appropriate behaviour.

Dentistry

A total of 13 articles were identified; 7 concerned children and 6 adults. One study was conducted in Canada and one in Denmark; the rest were from the USA.

Concerning children, the main goal was to reduce fear and encourage appropriate behaviour in children (a) making their first visit to the dentist (two studies), and (b) who were previously identified to be highly fearful (five studies).

The two studies in which attempts were made to reduce fear among children making their first visit to the dentist did not report positive results. However, this may be that the children were not screened for initial fearfulness, and it seems unlikely that the children who participated were fearful at all!

The remaining five studies are concerned with children who show excessive fear when visiting the dentist. These children represent a real problem from the point of view of the dentist; excessive anxiety making it difficult to perform the necessary treatment effectively; they are time-consuming and may create tension for other patients in the clinic as well as add to the stress of the professionals' working day. A method that effectively reduces anxiety and improves behaviour would therefore be generally valuable. Fearful children are generally first identified (usually through the Dental Anxiety Scale (Corah, 1969).

Without exception, workers in this area have taken the social learning model as their basic theoretical approach. However, the findings are disappointing. No differences were found between a video and a pre-treatment clinic visit (1), between a video presented as part of the general school curriculum *v.* in the dentist's office (2), or between a live *v.* video presentation (4). Only two studies reported more positive effects. The first (7) found that a coping video was more successful in reducing anxiety compared with a mastery model. The second (6) compared a mastery against a coping video. Neither was more effective in reducing anxiety or improving behaviour. However, both kinds of video were associated with improved behaviour and less anxiety compared with a placebo tape.

A major problem is that no study seems to have successfully identified children who were genuinely and excessively fearful in the dental setting (3, 4).

In *adult* work, four studies were concerned to reduce anxiety. One study had a specific goal of encouraging realistic expectations regarding false dentures and one study was intended to improve toothbrushing/plaque removal skills.

Again most studies have been concerned with the use of video to reduce dental anxiety. In this they have achieved little success. Two studies had more specific aims. One (9) attempted to change patients' expectations about dentures, pointing out that people were often quite unrealistic and non-accepting of problems they might experience with dentures. A specially prepared video describing difficulties likely to be experienced had no effect on patients' expectations. Another (11) compared the value of personal supervision with a video when teaching plaque removal. There were no differences between the methods regardless of whether subjects were genuine patients or laboratory technicians.

The studies involving children, and several involving adults, are all based on social learning theory. However, the general lack of success can probably be attributed to poor methodology and initial selection of samples as much as to any inadequacies of the theory itself. The poor results from these studies stand in sharp contrast to the success with which social learning theory has been used to guide work concerned with preparing children (and to a lesser extent adults) for general surgery. However, some results support our findings in other areas. First, multi-component packages rather than a video alone are potentially more useful (2). Second, the child's age and experience appears to interact with the intervention in determining the success of modelling videos (7).

Screening

Seven studies were identified. Of these, four were from the USA, 2 from Australia and 1 from the UK. Three studies used an after-only design, one a before–after without control and 2 used a before–after with control. One study (7) involved a larger survey.

While it is usually assumed that it is relatively straightforward to encourage middle-class or health conscious individuals to take part in screening programmes, it is acknowledged to be more difficult to encourage participation of people from socially disadvantaged backgrounds and/or with lower educational attainments. In some cases, these are also the people who are in fact at greater risk. Promotion of screening to minority ethnic groups can also pose special challenges. Recognition of this can be found in three of the studies. One of these (2) attempted to educate high-school girls from ethnic backgrounds to be aware of the potential value of *breast-screening*. This study did not involve a formal evaluation, but in that the girls said they would encourage their mothers and grandmothers to participate might be considered to be successful. Two other studies also reported success in encouraging women from ethnic (5) or lower educational backgrounds (6) to participate, both for *cervical screening*.

Study 5 is exemplary in the efforts that were made to develop videos suitable for an ethnic minority population. Their study also demonstrates that either videos or personal contact can be used to improve screening uptake (in comparison with simple distribution of informational leaflets). The videos were brief (5 minutes), informationally based and were well received by the target population (72 per cent made favourable comments). Outcome was measured in terms of screening uptake. At 2 or 4 months following the video, 47 per cent or 30 per cent (respectively) of women had attended for screening. There were no measures of attitude or knowledge included in the evaluation so it is not clear how far, if at all, the video was influential over wider areas of health behaviour, or had any repercussions for the health of the family more generally. However, the incidence of uptake was relatively impressive, especially given the assumed reluctance of this population to attend for screening.

An Australian study (6) used the Health Belief Model to guide decisions about the content of the video and outcome measures. Women were recruited from their workplace. There was a wide age range (19–63 years). Appropriateness of the model was achieved by producing two comparable videos; one being narrated by a young woman and one by an older woman. There was an increase in both knowledge and awareness of risks following the video. The authors also identified the major barriers to participation (embarrassment, concern about physical discomfort and worry about results). The video was seen to be successful in terms of behaviour; 34 per cent attended for screening within the follow-up period (5 weeks). Against this, there was a large attrition rate; the questionnaire was possibly too lengthy for the population studied, largely factory workers. While the video itself appeared useful, the value of the Health Belief Model was questioned. Variables related to the Health Belief Model (perceived severity, barriers, etc.) were not associated with the behaviours observed.

Personality differences in response to videos differing in degree of threat are examined in another Australian study (4). While concerned with acceptability of a test to detect lung cancer, the main focus of interest was the predictive value of a personality measure (*repression–sensitisation*) in combination with level of threat (high, medium or low) in the experimental video. The authors argue that *sensitisers* (those who intellectualise information) are more likely to respond to a health information video regardless of content, compared with *repressors* (those who characteristically deny or repress threatening information). As would be predicted, there was a trend for repressors to be more responsive to low rather than high threat information. Given its artificial nature, it is not clear how relevant these findings are to real-life situations.

Information which emphasises the risks of *not* screening appears more persuasive than information which focuses on the benefits of being screened (1). This was demonstrated in a well executed study in which take-up rates for mammography screening were greater where individuals watched a 'loss framed' video over those who watched a 'gain framed' video.

This area is likely to become increasingly important given the recent advances in human genetics and opportunities which arise to screen for a variety of conditions. It is important that psychological work keeps pace with developments in medicine and clinical practice; we may otherwise expect to see a large number of simplistic studies which fail to deal systematically with the range of psychological issues which need to be addressed. In this regard, the study by Fisher (3) which compared the value of video against personal counselling following screening may represent one direction for future work. In this area, it is not enough to increase participation in screening programmes. Consideration also needs to be given to the resulting psychological needs of the individual and family. Fisher raises the question that some of these needs may be met by use of video, but much more careful work is needed before widescale adoption of this method is seen to be appropriate.

Patient education

We identified 22 articles concerned with patient education. Of these, specific illnesses included *asthma, renal disease, diabetes, cardiac conditions* and *miscellaneous* (including hypertension). Videos have most commonly been used to inform patients about their disease or its management (fifteen studies), with a lesser emphasis on reducing anxiety or encouraging positive attitudes (seven studies). Attempts to modify behaviour have also been reported, with outcome assessed either by observation (seven studies) or self-report (four studies). Only two studies have attempted to document changes in symptomatology following intervention.

Either alone or as part of an intervention package, there is evidence that videos can be useful in this context. Of the fifteen studies which assessed knowledge, ten reported benefits and only one study concluded that no benefits occurred. All studies which used observation ratings of behaviour reported benefits while one of the four studies involving self-reported behaviour change reported positive effects. There was less consensus regarding impact on mood or anxiety; one study reported no positive effects.

Of the three papers concerned with asthma, one involved young children (1). This paper attempted to improve self-management skills, and is especially commendable in working with very young children (2–5 years). The other two papers involved adults and also focused on knowledge.

In the diabetes studies, only one successfully demonstrated any effects on self-care (8). This suggests an improvement in self-management among adolescent girls (but not adolescent boys or younger children). Small sample size and lack of support from other studies or theoretical rationale limits acceptability of this finding. There is evidence for the usefulness of video in teaching adolescents to measure their own blood pressure (16). Together these suggest some value in using video to teach self-care, at least in adolescent samples.

Considering other criteria, other studies conclude that there is no advantage in use of video over lecture, but video is cheaper (12); and that, when used as part of a package, videos can be useful in improving attendance (17).

*There is a disappointing emphasis on using video to increase knowledge rather than effect improved self-management. Despite the fact that some established scales are available to assess knowledge (at least in diabetes, for review see Bradley, 1994), studies in this area tend to rely on development of ad hoc measures to suit their own purposes. This means there is no comparability with other video studies, or with interventions involving other media. More importantly, it is not clear how gains in **knowledge** may translate to more practical self-care skills.*

Parenting

We identified 11 studies; 7 concerned with pregnancy and labour, and the remaining 4 concerned with parenting during the neonatal/infant period. Research concerned with pregnancy and labour has focused on issues of improving knowledge during pregnancy, making parents aware of the risks of premature labour and aware of signs of premature labour. Two studies focused on attempts to reduce pain during labour. The aims of the four studies about parenting were to improve parenting skills, with some focus on high-risk groups. (One study (11) targeted Vietnamese women in Australia and one study (9) targeted adolescent mothers.)

All but one study included appropriate samples for the question (i.e. pregnant or new mothers). Study 6 used female undergraduate subjects in an attempt to simulate labour pain. While competent methodologically, it is not at all clear that this work is relevant for samples experiencing actual labour pain.

Two studies suggest a positive impact of video (5 and 6). In other cases, there was either no comparison made or the video was used as part of a package. It should be noted however that neither of the apparently successful videos was appropriate in other ways. Study 6 involved female undergraduate subjects who were asked to participate in a project in which labour pain was artificially suggested (none of the subjects was pregnant). Study 5 involved professionals concerned in policy-making in deprived areas. Although professionals subsequently reported being more aware of the problems of prematurity, and this awareness was more pronounced in those watching a video compared with those hearing a lecture, there were no behavioural measures and it is not clear how they intended to make changes in policy and professional practice.

It must be concluded therefore that, especially when combined with additional forms of intervention, the video can be useful in giving information to expectant and new parents. This conclusion has to be tempered by awareness of the inadequacy of research in the area. No study was identified that could be said to achieve basic methodological acceptability. Although it might be expected that video could be employed usefully with high-risk mothers (whether these are adolescents or from deprived backgrounds) there was little attempt to do this. None of the above included fathers in their interventions.

4. An evaluation of the social learning approach

Identification of studies based on social learning

The extent to which interventions were based on social learning theories (including life/social skills, inoculation and the original Social Learning Theory) varied between the different areas reviewed. These differences reflect particularly the extent to which the subjects involved are children. In some sections (e.g. 'Dentistry') all articles involving children are based on social learning models while none of the articles involving adults use this approach. This is despite the fact that the aim of both types of work is very similar (to reduce fear and anxiety).

Of the six studies in 'AIDS', only two (16, 17) involved a simple comparison between a video and no intervention, but did suggest that the group who viewed a video was subsequently better in complying with treatment compared with the no-intervention controls. Study 14 involved five comparisons but reported no differences; the authors suggest that all participants were practising safe sex beforehand. Three studies (5, 6, 10) are more interesting in that all involved comparisons between simple modelling videos and additional skills training or rehearsal. In all cases, the combined effects appeared most successful.

For 'Alcohol', we identified 9 studies. One study (10) suggests a simple advantage of video by itself over no-treatment control. Again there is evidence that the modelling video plus rehearsal is most effective (3, 4, 7, 8, 9).

For 'Smoking', of the 15 articles identified, there is evidence that any intervention is better than no intervention (1, 6, 7, 15, 19, 21). There is mixed evidence regarding the value of model similarity. Study 10 finds no specific advantage for a peer-led intervention over an adult-led one. However, in study 15, better results were obtained for a video plus peer leader compared with the video alone.

Three articles were identified in the 'Nutrition' literature (8, 9, 10). However, all three studies were by the same authors, and overlap considerably.

In 'Miscellaneous health promotion', one study (5) suggested that a video alone was better than standard procedures in recruiting young people to donate blood. Both of the others suggest the value of incorporating feedback/rehearsal with the video.

In the 'Preparation for surgery' literature, social learning theory is used extensively in work with children, but much less so in work with adults. In many ways, this is the most important area in which to assess the value of the social learning approach, in that a series of studies has been conducted and efforts have been made to test some of the main assumptions of the theory. As a consequence, systematic attempts have been reported to determine the importance of other variables on the success of interventions (e.g. age, previous experience or model similarity). A number of studies, however, failed to demonstrate the superiority of modelling videos (1, 3, 6, 8, 20). This is variously attributed to lack of model similarity, or previous hospital experience or lack of initial anxiety; these explanations are however post hoc and unsatisfactory.

For 'Dentistry', 7 of the 13 articles are based on children and all 7 used social learning models. None of the adult studies is based on social learning. Again there are some negative findings. No effects are reported in studies 1, 3, or 4.

None of the 'Screening' articles used social learning methods. This may reflect a lack of focus on children as subjects.

The number of studies in 'Patient education' based on social learning is also low, and those that were identified did tend to involve children. All four studies report positive findings associated with the approach.

Again the number of relevant studies in 'Parenting' is low. Study 9 involved teenage mothers and appears to be especially successful in promoting appropriate mothering in the group.

Percentage of studies based on social learning by area

AIDS	22
Alcohol	53
Drugs	63
Smoking	54
Nutrition	38
Miscellaneous health	25
Surgery	55
Dentistry	54
Screening	0
Patient education	18
Parenting	18

Model similarity

Evidence for the importance of model similarity is far from conclusive. A same sex model was more successful than an opposite sex model in encouraging appropriate attitudes to drink ('Alcohol' 1). A peer leader in addition to a modelling video was reported to be better than the video alone in inhibiting take-up of cigarette smoking ('Smoking' 15). In the surgery area, the importance of model similarity has been stressed ('Preparation for surgery' 1, 4).

Conclusions

In evaluating the social learning approach, it may therefore be important to consider the question in relation to (i) chronological age and (ii) the specific area being investigated. It is possible to point to some successful studies involving children or adolescents; this is less easy to do when considering the work based on adults. In each area reviewed, some successful studies can be identified. However, in preparation for surgery and dentistry particularly, despite the fact that social learning has been a dominant approach, a good proportion of studies have failed to report positive effects.

Some of the key issues in social learning theory (model similarity, opportunity to rehearse the behaviours modelled, the relative merits of coping versus mastery models) have received very little systematic investigation and tend to be reported almost incidentally. This probably reflects the interests of most workers in this area. Social learning theory is used as a tool to investigate the key question, which is related to the healthcare issue. Other work which relates to more theoretical questions about the processes through which the methods operate is considered in more experimental studies, the results of which tend not to have informed developments in the applied area.

It is perhaps important to bear in mind the original limitations of social learning theory as put forward by Bandura (1977). To the extent that the theory explicitly stated that, in order to promote effective behaviour change, four subprocesses needed to be defined (attention, encoding, motor skills and rehearsal or feedback), it must be concluded that few studies have involved fair assessments of the value of the theory. Mere presentation is not sufficient. The development of video must not take place in a vacuum, and should only be considered when part of a coherent package, which incorporates opportunities for encoding, rehearsal and feedback.

5. Summary and conclusions

Overall evaluation

Considering the studies across all eleven different areas, we are forced to conclude that many provide little or no positive evidence for the effectiveness of video or of any health education intervention of which video forms a part. Even where positive findings are claimed, a number of studies suffer from flaws in the design which render any apparent effect untrustworthy.

However, it is also very clear that a large number of these so-called 'evaluations' have been poorly conducted and fall far short of the standards one would normally expect of scientific research publications. Evaluations can yield negative results, among other reasons because of a lack of power (small sample size) and inappropriate outcome measures. In other words, the main faults may sometimes be associated with the conduct of the evaluation rather than the content of the intervention itself. However, our impression is that many of the interventions associated with poorly conducted evaluations did indeed fail because they were poorly planned and delivered in the first place. Many seemed to lack any clear notion of what effects they expected to find or of the processes by which these effects might be brought about.

Often the interventions were presented to a target group without any evidence that they had been developed with that group so as to match the content of any programme to the real concerns of that group.

Much of this work therefore tells us little about the potential effectiveness of video in different areas of health education. In considering this question, more can be learned from the minority of well-designed evaluations which yield more reliable (and sometimes encouraging) results.

The specific advantages of video

The question of the effectiveness of video is narrower than the question of the effectiveness of health education in general. As has been remarked upon throughout this review, many interventions – including many of the more successful ones – have used video in combination with other procedures. The distinctive effectiveness of video in the absence of anything else has not been the question addressed by the evaluations and for many practical purposes it is perhaps not the most important question to ask anyway, since there is no suggestion that video, however successful, should replace all other forms of health education.

Nonetheless, taking the narrower question as posed, the place to start is to ask what it is that video can do that other media can do less easily. The answer is simple, but has important implications.

Video can show things

From this it follows that video is likely to be most effective when there is something worth showing. This comes out clearly from the studies reviewed. Video has demonstrable advantages when used to present:

1. models of specific behaviours to be imitated and rehearsed
2. information in an appealing form
3. information about the damaging consequences of unhealthy behaviour.

These advantages will be considered in turn.

1. Models of specific behaviours to be imitated and rehearsed

A major advantage of video is the facility to present, in a standard and controlled way, models of specific behaviours to be imitated and rehearsed. The most successful interventions are those employing a well-conceived version of behavioural modelling, either to teach specific actions or to reduce anxiety among patients undergoing medical procedures, although (particularly in the latter case) there are a number of studies that fail to find positive effects. We can conclude, therefore, that a social learning/modelling perspective increases the chances of a successful intervention but, even here, success is far from guaranteed.

It is important to remember that, according to social learning theory, mere presentation of a model for imitation is not predicted to produce behaviour change. The information must be properly attended to and encoded and the individual must have the skills to imitate the model and receive reinforcement and feedback to sustain successful imitation. Failure to satisfy these requirements may be one reason why not all modelling interventions appear to work, but there are almost certainly other reasons which are less easy to identify from the published studies. We suspect that some interventions seek to 'impose' models of health behaviour for imitation with insufficient prior consideration of their appropriateness or credibility within particular social contexts or for particular target groups. Under such circumstances, recommended actions may not be imitated because of their 'lack of fit' with other social norms or valued activities. Conversely, programmes based on careful pre-testing, for example for cultural appropriateness, may avoid such pitfalls.

These suggestions are tentative and impressionistic, since relevant details of both programme development and effectiveness are rarely reported. Even so, a number of studies in our review highlight the value of programmes which are developed with sensitivity to the cultural context within which they are to be applied. There are some excellent examples of the use of video in community-based interventions in inner cities and with ethnic minorities. O'Donnell *et al.* (1994) describe the importance of qualitative research in the development stage of a programme aimed at the reduction of AIDS and STDs among inner-city Hispanics in New York City. Cultural appropriateness again is something that depends on more than good intentions. It depends on formative research.

2. Information in an appealing form

Presentation of information through video may be appealing to special groups that are of particular importance for health education: young children and people with lower socio-economic status and educational attainments. This is consistent with the notion that relevant health messages must be attended to and encoded if they are to produce behavioural change. Social learning theory states this as an explicit assumption, but it is also implicit in other approaches, including more systematic versions of an 'informational' approach. However, the mere 'acceptability' of a video presentation should not be regarded as evidence of actual or even probable effectiveness.

3. Information about the damaging consequences of unhealthy behaviour

Few would deny that an important responsibility of health education is to present information about the damaging consequences of unhealthy behaviour and/or the benefits of healthy behaviour. Unless one can be certain that this knowledge is already widely shared, the debate is not so much over whether to present such information, but how. Through video, relevant information can often be communicated in a memorable, personally involving and even (sometimes) shocking way. Video allows such messages to be conveyed through dramatic narrative and/or through striking visual imagery. This suggestion runs counter to one of the most widespread examples of 'received wisdom' in this area – that a high level of fear-arousal is counterproductive. It is important when considering this issue to distinguish two questions. First, what is the relationship between levels of fear-arousal and behavioural motivation? Second, what factors may account for the fact that individuals do not always change their behaviour, even when fearful of the health risks they currently run?

The relationship between fear and behavioural change

With respect to the first question, the debate dates back to an early experimental study by Janis and Feshbach (1953), which appeared to show that a shocking film about dental disease produced less improvement in toothbrushing than a milder film. Although the communications did not in fact produce significant differences in levels of reported fear, this exceptional study was taken as the basis for elaborate theory-building (e.g. Janis, 1967) to account for a supposed curvilinear relationship between fear and behaviour change, with maximum effectiveness at moderate levels of fear. In fact, the generality of empirical findings in this area does not support this prediction but rather points to a monotonic relationship between fear and change in intention and/or behaviour (see Sutton, 1982, 1992, for reviews).

Put simply, fear is a powerful motivator for behaviour change and more fear produces more motivation.

What other factors should be considered?

On the other hand, many of the same studies that demonstrate an effect of fear also show other (more cognitive) factors to be important. Among these, belief in one's ability to take suitable protective action seems to be very important. This in turn may be influenced by straightforward procedural knowledge about how to achieve such self-protection. Health messages that call for rather demanding forms of behavioural or lifestyle change may sometimes appear to be less effective for reasons unrelated to how much fear they produce. Another problem can occur if people regard a health message as irrelevant to themselves. Extreme health costs may be seen as linked only to extreme forms of risk-taking. Individuals who consider themselves as only moderate risk-takers (e.g. 'light' smokers, 'social' drinkers, etc.) might differentiate themselves from the target characters in a 'shock-horror' film. However, if they do so, they will be less likely to experience fear anyway, so this is really an argument for more convincing script-writing rather than against the principle of fear-arousal as such.

None of this settles the ethical question of whether or not health educators *should* seek to frighten their target audience (least of all in contexts where the precise relationship between behaviour and disease is uncertain). Nor does it remove the need to make a judgement whether, in any given situation, the intended audience is more lacking in motivation to change their behaviour or in knowledge about how to go about it (which is something that other kinds of video also might provide). There is also the issue of whether one is seeking to deter those not yet engaging in a risk behaviour or to change the behaviour of those who have already adopted a less healthy lifestyle. There is still much sense in the view that just frightening people is (often) not enough. Even so, the capacity of individuals to play down their levels of personal risk can be considerable.

Judicious, credible, and factually sound use of fear-arousing information may be one way of combating such rationalisations.

Other advantages

There are other advantages that follow directly from the fact that videos not only use the visual medium but are recordings. An apparently underexploited feature of health education videos is that they can be taken away and shown on repeated occasions (but see 'Patient education' 2). More sophisticated use of video through interactive computer systems appears to be very promising as a means of providing people with the health information that they want. The few recent studies using such techniques report notable successes ('Parenting' 9; 'Nutrition' 8, 9, 10).

Potential pitfalls

Against these advantages, what may be some of the potential pitfalls? Possibly the most important is the fact that just screening a video does not mean that it will be watched or attended to. Those interventions which have simply had videos playing in the background in surgery waiting-rooms or supermarkets have consistently failed. Where television (and the need sometimes to ignore it) is so much a feature of everyday life, passive exposure is not enough. Active engagement is vital.

A second cautionary note is that dramatic narratives presented on video may need to choose a single story line in a way that might sometimes fail to do justice to the multiple ways in which health problems can arise ('Drugs' 2; 'Miscellaneous' 2).

There are other ways in which a video may not be obviously any worse than other media, but where there are no special advantages. Into this category would seem to fall videos that merely present lectures, exhortations or 'talking heads', or list facts that can be communicated in other ways. The cost-effectiveness of such interventions needs to be carefully examined. For some purposes, leaflets may often be cheaper to produce, but less effective if reading ability or linguistic competence is an issue. Much may also depend on the technical quality of the video (as opposed to just the content of the message) since this may affect how well it commands the attention of the audience, as well as on how it is distributed and where it is viewed.

Need for coordination between programme development and evaluation

We know from our own experience that very many health authorities and charities have for some time been developing their own videos on a variety of (sometimes overlapping) topics. For all we know, the quality of many of these may be excellent, but if they are not systematically evaluated, there is no way of telling if they have any effect. Our review suggests that only a minority of video-based interventions (at least in the UK) have been systematically evaluated, even at the most basic level of establishing the extent of their use.

Perhaps the single most important implication from this review is that too often there appears to be little coordination between the process of intervention programme development on the one hand and the process of evaluation on the other.

Evaluation research does require some prior commitment of funds, but one suspects very much less than is committed to the video productions themselves. There is also the important point that the evaluation process is not something which can be simply 'tagged on' at the end, like some kind of afterthought.

Particularly with national campaigns, researchers may sometimes be asked to evaluate interventions that are already under way, so that the possibility of obtaining necessary baseline measures or a proper control group is denied to them.

A built-in plan for evaluation is thus very much part of essential good practice for programme development. The most successful studies in this review tend to be those where the planning of the intervention and the planning of the evaluation go hand-in-hand.

Why might the importance of a research element in programme development and evaluation not be more widely acknowledged? The answer seems to lie in the atheoretical nature of much of this activity. The findings of our review are absolutely clear on this point.

Interventions without a clear theoretical rationale almost always fail or achieve only a semblance of success that disappears when submitted to critical examination.

They do not know precisely what they are trying to change, or by what means, or how to tell if they have succeeded. By contrast, an encouraging proportion of theoretically-based interventions actually succeed in changing health attitudes and behaviour, albeit to greater extents in some domains than others. Even where such interventions are less successful, it is easier to infer where things went wrong. Often this seems to be because the behaviours being modelled or messages being communicated are not precisely specified or perceived as relevant to the health decisions in hand.

This conclusion – that interventions need a theoretical base – is in many ways more important than the choice of which theory to use. This may sound slightly heretical, since the goal of much academic research is to establish the superiority of one kind of theoretical account over another. Even so, many of the factors that give interventions a better chance of success are shared in common by a broad range of theoretical approaches. These include (ideally) a disciplined approach to the statement of hypotheses, clear operational definition of specified variables, recognition of the need for reliable measurement and anticipation of the need for appropriate control and comparison conditions. At a more conceptual level, there is also much common ground between many of the more widely used theories in terms of their underlying assumptions. Deliberate adoption of a specific conceptual and methodological approach (or of a combination of approaches) gives research projects a focus; one can see what the researchers were trying to do, how and why. Conversely, studies that lack such focus are also difficult to locate in terms of their relationships to previous research. Even where their results appear promising, they run the risk of merely reinventing the wheel.

Future directions

1. Videos have a potential role to play in a variety of healthcare settings. However, realistic attention needs to be paid to their limitations. Simply showing a video is not enough, but it is important that the video is an integral part of any package. In designing any intervention package, consideration needs to be given to those aspects which can best be communicated through video (e.g. demonstrations) while also recognising those aspects that cannot successfully be portrayed by video.

2. The range of situations that have been addressed in the research reviewed does not represent the full range of issues to which video might be expected to contribute. Researchers need to be aware of innovations in medical practice which open new avenues of work. Videos may be particularly useful in hospitals for helping families understand a relative's illness and teaching them specific aspects of medical care that they could usefully perform. For example, a study supported by the Dutch Heart Foundation is concerned with the fact that heart attacks often occur at home, perhaps at night, when immediate action is necessary by relatives. A study is under way to teach relatives resuscitation procedures and appears to show some success following a video teaching package. This work also highlights the limitations of videos which take a purely educational stance, in that relatives report an increase in anxiety and concern.

3. Most work is still directed at certain populations, especially school-aged children and adults, rather than younger children or the elderly. Videos are likely to be especially useful for special groups. (Even pre-school children have been able to learn to use their own inhaler when shown an appropriate video; 'Patient education' 3). The elderly too may benefit from the opportunities for repeated viewing which is possible using video, while being reluctant to take too much professional time. Too much work in hospital settings has however focused on general issues of preparation for surgery, for example, while also employing very general outcome measures. There are many practical problems in healthcare settings (e.g. teaching people with diabetes to recognise foot problems and how to deal with them; teaching parents of children with leukaemia how to clean the Hickman line at home). Helping patients and relatives to learn about these issues may lead to more home-based care, which in turn could mean greater home- rather than hospital-based care (an advantage to both the NHS and patients). It is not however appropriate to use videos in all circumstances. Although the literature on preparing children for surgery is more comprehensive than others, it is limited in terms of practical value. Most work has been conducted with older children, while it is in fact younger children who present the most difficulties in the clinic. The solution has to be integrated work which addresses real questions, while at the same time giving adequate consideration to issues of sampling and outcome assessment. Greater collaboration between medical staff and social scientists is essential.

Appendices

Appendix A. The main theoretical approaches

The studies included in this review are based on a variety of theoretical approaches, the most important of which are summarised below.

Informational approaches

A large number of studies have been classified as 'informational'. At best, these are based on a structured consideration of what facts need to be communicated to the public or patients concerning a specific issue, and adopt the straightforward goal of improving knowledge. More often, studies in this category are essentially atheoretical, and offer relatively general health information and exhortations in the hope that this may influence knowledge, attitudes and behaviour.

The Health Belief Model

The Health Belief Model (HBM) was originally proposed by Rosenstock (1966) in order to explain preventive behaviours such as check-ups and immunisation. It was extended by Becker (1974) to apply to a broad range of self-protective activities. According to the model, there are four major types of subjective judgements or beliefs that influence the likelihood of taking action in a health-related context:

(a) perceived susceptibility (the likelihood of personally contracting the disease);

(b) perceived seriousness (severity) of the disease ((a) and (b) together contribute to 'perceived threat');

(c) perceived benefits of the preventive action; and

(d) perceived barriers to preventive action.

Although more a listing of important predictor variables than a model of causal processes, the HBM has proved relatively useful in a range of contexts. Particularly helpful is the attention paid to 'perceived barriers', which offers a possible way of making sense of apparent discrepancies between health attitudes and behaviours.

Decision-making approaches

In all of these, a crucial element is the individual's calculation of the probability of certain consequences attendant on performing or not performing a given action. Economists would recognise this as an instance of 'subjective expected utility' (SEU). There is a strong emphasis on 'rationality' (doing whatever produces the most desired consequences), but there is also a realisation that some individuals may find unhealthy activities very desirable for other reasons, and that they may not always calculate consequences in an unbiased way. A widely-used model is the *Theory of Reasoned Action* (Ajzen and Fishbein, 1980), which predicts behavioural intention from a combination of 'attitude' (conceived of as an overall evaluation based on SEU-type beliefs about consequences) and 'subjective norm' (beliefs about how one's behaviour will be evaluated by significant others). A recent revision, the *Theory of Planned Behaviour* (Ajzen, 1991) adds 'perceived behavioural control' as a predictor of intention.

Among approaches that emphasise biases in this 'rational' decision-making process are Weinstein's (1983) work on *optimistic bias* (which states that individuals are likely to rate their personal susceptibility to a range of mishaps as less than that of other people) and *Prospect Theory* (Kahneman and Tversky, 1979). The latter predicts that people are 'risk-averse' for gains, i.e. will prefer to take a sure profit than opt for an uncertain but larger gain, but that they are 'risk-seeking' for losses, i.e. they will prefer to gamble than accept a sure loss (hence, perhaps, Nick Leeson and the collapse of Barings). Sometimes the same probabilities can be 'framed' with reference to gaining positive outcomes (e.g. staying healthy) as opposed to averting negative outcomes (e.g. avoiding illness).

However, it is debatable whether such effects are really the consequence of motivational factors, or rather of differential exposure to positive and negative feedback as a consequence of action. For instance, standard theories of reinforcement learning (which are part of the basis for *Social Learning Theory*, see below) predict that people will tend to repeat actions which lead to gains or 'rewards', and avoid actions found in the past to lead to losses or 'punishments'. This leads not only to a modification of behaviour, but to an uneven sampling of contingencies in the environment. When considering gains, choices that lead only rarely to gains (however large) are less likely (in the short term) to be rewarded and hence repeated than choices associated with certain benefits. Likewise, in the context of losses, riskier choices may, for a while, escape any 'punishment' whatsoever and so will be less likely to be avoided than those that always result in a (smaller) loss (see March, 1996). Although this evidently cannot account for people's preparedness either to gamble on lotteries or to buy insurance, it may be relevant that promotion of both such activities seems to involve considerable emphasis on the gains and losses which *other people* have experienced.

Social learning theory

Social learning theory refers to a class of inter-connected approaches that derives from general psychological learning theory, adapted so as to take account of some of the complexities of human social behaviour. At base, the theory is concerned with the acquisition of behaviours. The main processes of learning, or behaviour acquisition are *association, reinforcement (reward), practice and imitation.* Individuals also acquire expectancies about the consequences of their actions and about their own ability to perform particular tasks or achieve particular goals. The terms 'locus of control' and 'self-efficacy' are used to refer to people's general or more specific expectancies in their ability to control important events or to achieve certain goals. 'Behavioural efficacy', like 'perceived behavioural control' (Ajzen, 1991) refers to confidence in one's ability to carry out a particular behaviour (giving up cigarettes, for example). The important assumption of social learning theory is that these expectancies are learned through past successes and failures. This in turn is sometimes taken to imply that the acquisition of more general social competence or 'life skills' can lead to higher self-esteem and more efficacious coping with stressful or challenging situations.

The most common form of intervention based on social learning theory is that of *modelling*, for instance when a target group is shown an example of a desired form of behaviour to imitate. What is often forgotten (and has been in many of the studies to be described) is that a basic assumption of social learning theory is that the mere presentation of a model would never suffice to produce a sustained change in behaviour. Bandura (1977) identified four subprocesses necessary for imitation to occur. First, the observer must *attend* to the critical modelling behaviour. Second, the observed behaviour must be *encoded* (through visual imagery and verbal labelling, sustained by cognitive rehearsal) in such a way that the relevant information can later be retrieved from memory so as to guide behaviour when the model is no longer present. Third, the observer must have the *motor skills* to reproduce the modelled behaviours (this may be relevant to the imitation of physical exercise, for instance, or self-care among the elderly). Fourth, although modelled behaviour can be initially acquired through observation alone, *reinforcement* is necessary for the behaviour to be actually performed and for such performance to persist. One of the best ways of ensuring that these subprocesses are all brought into play is to combine a modelling presentation with sessions in which participants *rehearse* the desired behaviours and receive *feedback* (i.e. reinforcement) on the quality of their performance.

These core ideas have been developed in a number of different directions. One of the most important for this review is the *social/life-skills* approach. This sets itself the ambitious goal of helping adolescents to acquire the cognitive and interpersonal skills and broader self-awareness that will allow them to cope confidently with stresses in general and unwanted social pressures in particular. A narrower aim is to teach specific strategies to resist such pressures (e.g. to refuse an offer of an unwanted drug or cigarette) and defend oneself against others' attempts at persuasion. This approach is often combined with McGuire's (1964) *inoculation theory*, which proposes that a way to make someone's attitude more resistant to change is to present them with weak arguments on the other side, against which counter-arguments can be readily found and rehearsed.

Stages of change

Another general framework specifically developed with respect to smoking cessation and the treatment of addictive behaviours is the 'stages of change' model of Prochaska and DiClemente (1983). This proposes that individuals pass through a sequence of relatively discrete stages on the path to cessation or recovery from addiction. During the *precontemplation* stage, smokers (etc.) give no active consideration to the question of quitting or cutting down. During the *contemplation* stage, they consider quitting, and may resolve to do so, but not necessarily set a date for their attempt. Next, during the *action* stage, they will actually attempt to quit or cut down. (Recent applications of the model include a *preparation* stage between contemplation and action, but the operational definition of this extra stage has attracted criticism, since it requires individuals to have failed in a recent cessation attempt.) If successful at the action stage, individuals then pass to the *maintenance* stage, where the issue is one of sustaining abstinence and avoiding relapse.

Although basically a descriptive rather than explanatory model, this approach alerts one to the possibility that the success or failure of any intervention may depend on the 'stage' of the target group. For example, a programme designed to motivate people to adopt a healthier lifestyle may be most effective if the target group is at the 'precontemplation' stage and needs to be moved towards 'contemplation'. On the other hand, as individuals move towards or into the 'action' stage, they may derive more benefit from advice on how to give up smoking, lose weight, or whatever. The main difficulty seems to be one of validating such stage distinctions independently of the behavioural changes that are assumed to follow from them, particularly since the time individuals spend within any stage can be highly variable. One also needs to allow for regression to previous stages either temporarily (e.g. as a result of mood) or more permanently (e.g. as a result of failed attempts at cessation). Progression through stages may thus be more complex than the simple sequence suggests.

Other theories

There are other theories that make important predictions about attitude and behaviour change, but few of these feature in the studies to be reviewed. A small number of studies represent the long tradition of *personality* research which attempts to predict variations in behaviour and/or emotional reactions from independently identified dimensions of individual difference. More social psychological theories include *Attribution Theory*, which considers people's subjective explanations (attributions) for events, including their own behaviour and emotions. *Social Identity Theory* considers the subjective importance of people's group membership, and how this affects their reactions to outgroup members (who may sometimes include health communicators). It is disappointing how little of this research directly investigates the nature of relevant group and interpersonal processes, with only a small number prepared to consider even adolescent health education in relation to family contexts.

Appendix B. Details of the methodology

Databases used

The main databases used were PsychLIT, Medline and Unicorn (HEA). The educational resources database ERIC was also searched but mainly produced details of videos available for health education rather than reports of evaluations of the effectiveness of any video. PsychLIT in particular appears extensive and reliable for this topic when appropriately interrogated. Even so, we found a few additional articles by handsearching key journals. There is therefore the possibility that a limited number of relevant articles in other journals were also missed, presumably because of the manner in which they were entered into the databases.

It should be noted that PsychLIT does not have an inbuilt thesaurus or controlled vocabulary such as that provided by Mesh headings in Medline. Indeed, across the range of journals and disciplines surveyed in this review, there was no single set of subject headings from which key words could be selected.

Keywords used

The keywords used were as follows:

film/movie/video (PsychLIT) *or* videorecording (Medline)

and

AIDS/HIV
asthma
breast self-examination
cancer
catheterisation
compliance
dental/oral care/health
diabetes
diet/nutritition/eating disorders
drinking/alcohol
drug/drug abuse prevention/drug education
exercise/sport
family knowledge/family support
gastroenterology
health education
health knowledge

health promotion
heart disease/coronary disease/cardiovascular disease/angioplasty
hypertension
medical treatment/medical procedure/health care
patient education
perinatal/prenatal/pregnancy
prevention
(mass) screening
smoking
surgery/anxiety.

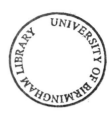

Inclusion and exclusion criteria

From these searches, a total of 264 articles were initially identified. Of these, 32 were excluded on the basis of the published abstracts, principally because it was apparent that the article did not report any findings relating to the effectiveness of video in health education. From the 232 articles then assembled, a further 57 were excluded on the basis of a full reading, leaving 175. Again, the most common reason was that no evaluation of video effectiveness was reported. In many cases, the paper merely described the content of video-based intervention programmes without providing evidence of effectiveness. Hence, our *main exclusion criterion* was a failure to report any *attempt* at an evaluation of video, either by itself or as part of a more general evaluation.

In a few other cases, video was used but not as part of a relevant intervention. For instance, subjects might be presented with stimulus material via video as part of an experimental study on forming impressions of a speaker's personality or credibility (although a few of these are retained where they are relevant to processes determining the relative effectiveness of different kinds of messages or presentations). A few other papers were excluded because they describe findings also reported or summarised in another article by the same authors. 'Position papers' which did not report specific findings were also excluded. Previous review articles (of which there are very few) are cited in this report, along with the occasional reference to work not involving videos, but are not included in the tabulations.

It is less easy to be specific about the *inclusion criteria* employed, apart from simply stating that any study, published in an English language journal and *claiming* to evaluate any form of health education involving video, was presumed to qualify for inclusion. We are well aware that such a generous and all-embracing criterion would be inappropriate in many other contexts. We are dealing here with a literature that is extremely heterogeneous with respect both to the aims of the various interventions and to the methods employed to evaluate them. There is no single or simple consensus regarding the kind of *outcomes* that provide a valid indicator of effectiveness, since there is a diversity of views regarding the primary, or at any rate, proximal goals of health education itself. Should health education seek to inform or to persuade, to change attitudes or to change behaviour, to promote self-care or a greater use of medical services? The answer depends partly on the context, and partly also on the theoretical approach, if any, that the researchers adopt. It will also be evident that the researchers contributing to this literature have been trained in a variety of disciplines, where, to some extent, there may be different expectations concerning the acceptability of different kinds of *research designs*.

This methodological variety presented us with our main dilemma. We could have specified conventional criteria for soundness of experimental design (from a behavioural science perspective) and chosen simply to exclude all studies that we found wanting. However, this approach, if adopted here, would have led to serious difficulties. Firstly, as discussed in the report itself, relatively few of the studies we have reviewed would measure up to the more rigorous standards demanded of the leading journals in our own discipline. Thus, we would be left discussing a very small body of work. Secondly, because of this, the process would lack transparency, not least from the perspective of researchers and practitioners in other disciplines. We therefore chose instead to include all studies *claiming* to report an evaluation, and then comment on the soundness or otherwise of the designs employed within the text of our review.

Thirdly, while it is unfortunately the case that many of the studies included lack rigour as controlled evaluations, some nonetheless suggest lessons for future practice, for instance with respect to how the interventions themselves were developed. Fourthly, and related to this, it may be a better corrective from the point of view of future evaluation research to mention such studies and explain their faults, than simply not to mention them at all.

Limitations of the methodology

Effect size
This report attempts to draw generalisations on the basis of the studies reviewed in the different domains. Individual studies are identified for special mention, particularly if they are distinctive in their approach or yield instructive findings. However, the main impression that the reader may gain may merely be one of the number of articles that conform to certain criteria. For tabulation purposes, the unit of analysis is the

individual study, irrespective of the statistical size of any effects it reports. This review is therefore in no sense a meta-analysis (a technique for assessing the statistical reliability of an effect over a series of comparable studies). In fact, the diversity of designs and the variable methodological quality of this body of literature would mean that very few of the studies cited could be included in a formal meta-analysis.

'File drawer' bias

There is also a potential problem – common to all such reviews – which is sometimes termed the 'file drawer' bias. This refers to the presumption that authors may be less motivated to submit, and editors less inclined to accept, reports of negative findings for publication in academic journals. (Hence researchers' file drawers may contain numerous reports of 'failed' experiments.) The extent of any such bias in this instance is difficult to determine. Had we been dealing with a more narrowly defined topic, a possible strategy would have been to contact the key groups of researchers in the field with a view to identifying unpublished work. However, the diversity of the relevant literature precluded such an approach here (which would in any event have exceeded both the remit and resources of the contract). We are not dealing here with something comparable to clinical evaluations of a new treatment, conducted in a few easily identified centres. If we had chosen to contact some researchers but not others directly, this could have itself introduced a new source of bias. The fact that a high proportion of the literature is from North America should also be remembered.

In any event, it is difficult to regard this literature as one where there is an evident bias against the publication of statistically inconclusive results. Indeed, a large number of the reported findings are in fact negative with respect to outcome criteria relevant to this review. Nonetheless, it may be noted that, where negative findings are reported, authors look beyond the immediate analyses to justify publication. It is particularly in studies that report negative findings that anecdotal comments tend to appear suggesting that, notwithstanding the absence of a statistically reliable effect, the intervention was 'economical in terms of professional time' or 'acceptable' to a target audience.

Defining effectiveness

We are also faced with a major difficulty in defining 'effectiveness' or a 'positive effect'. As has been explained (a) many studies do not test for the distinctive effects of a video (let alone specific components of a video message); and (b) there is less than unanimity over the goals that any health education intervention should seek to achieve. For these reasons, we have attempted to derive the best indications, from the evidence available, of whether video can work. Although in some cases it will be possible to be more specific, in general such evidence will relate to the effectiveness of interventions including, or built upon, the use of video rather than to the impact of video per se.

Hence, in tabulating the findings of the different studies, we have adopted very lenient criteria for accepting a positive 'video effect'. Essentially, whenever any treatment including a video element shows an advantage on any outcome measure over another condition without a video (or with a video on another topic), we record this as a positive effect. In some cases (where the design involves a before–after comparison without a control), we may record as a positive effect the presence of an improvement in the same individuals, assumed by the authors to be attributable to the intervention, while recognising that the absence of a control group renders this conclusion uncertain. Where authors' claims of a positive impact are undermined by more serious design flaws, this is specifically noted.

Specific domains reviewed

The effectiveness of video with respect to the following domains was reviewed in terms of two broad categories comprising separate sections:

1. Health promotion and prevention (102 studies)

AIDS and sexually transmitted diseases
Alcohol
Drugs
Smoking
Nutrition
Miscellaneous health promotion and prevention

2. Healthcare settings (73 studies)

Preparation for surgery
Preparation for dentistry
Screening
Patient education
Parenting.

This classification (in combination with the classification of interventions below) differentiates studies with respect to issues such as the numbers of groups used and the timing of measures relative to any intervention, and hence point to the type of statistical analysis that would be appropriate. What it does not explicitly state is how individuals were assigned to different groups or experimental treatments. In clinical trials, the presumption is that individuals will be assigned to different treatment 'arms', or to active or placebic treatments, at random, using double-blind procedures wherever possible. The present context is somewhat different

Classification/evaluation criteria

Each study was separately classified, where appropriate, according to the following criteria (the separate coding forms for each study having been deposited with the HEA). All studies were coded by at least one of three coders, using the agreed coding scheme. Approximately 30 per cent of the studies were coded independently by two coders, with a small number of discrepancies in the initial stages prompting refinement of the coding categories. All such discrepancies were resolved by discussion.

Country:
Topic:
Other relevant areas:
Authors:
Title:
Reference:
Aim:
Study design:
Intervention group(s):
Control/comparison group(s):
Sample:
Age range:
Allocation:
Theoretical rationale:
Content of video:
Dependent measures:
    Manipulation checks, acceptability
    Knowledge
    Attitudes
    Behaviour
Mediating/subject variables included in design:
Comments on selection of dependent measures (reliability, rationale, etc.):
Timing of post-measures, follow-up(s):
Attrition rates at follow-up(s):
Analyses, results and conclusions:
Comments on analyses, results and conclusions.

Types of study design

The following main types of study design were identified.

A: **After only**

B: **Before–after** (i.e. repeated measures without control)

C: **Before–after with control**

D: **Solomon four-group**
    This is regarded as one of the best designs for evaluation of interventions, combining the extra power of design C with safeguards against the reactive influence of repeated testing. The four groups are:
    (i)   before measure – intervention – after measure
    (ii)   before measure – no intervention – after measure
    (iii) intervention – after measure only
    (iv) no intervention – after measure only.

E : **Other**

for various reasons. Although assessment of long-term behavioural change may (and, where possible, should) be accomplished without knowledge of the conditions to which individuals had been assigned, the interventions themselves typically cannot be given 'blind'. In other words, those delivering the interventions typically have to be aware what the interventions are.

A more difficult issue is that of random assignment to intervention or control conditions. There are several examples in this set of studies where greater attention by the researchers to the benefits of random-isation would have strengthened our confidence in the findings reported. Even so, practical considerations are also important. Many studies depend on volunteer samples, the representativeness of which may be uncertain. Others, notably those conducted in school settings, involve assignment of *groups* (e.g. school classes), not *individuals*, to different conditions. Since one of the possible benefits of video interventions is their potential for group administration, such a procedure makes good practical sense. However, it represents a departure from classical experimental design, especially if students within each class are considered as independent individuals for purposes of analysis. Another problem, when different classes within the same school are assigned to different conditions, is whether some 'contagion' might occur, through students and teachers discussing the different forms of intervention among themselves. However, designating different schools as experimental and control groups carries the risk of introducing other extrinsic sources of variation.

Appendix C. Table of studies

Key to abbreviations in tables

The tables summarising the studies within each domain contain the following abbreviations.

Column heading: Theoretical perspective
HBM   Health Belief Model
SEU   Subjective Expected Utility
SL   Social Learning
TPB   Theory of Planned Behaviour
TRA   Theory of Reasoned Action

Column heading: DES (design)
A   After only
B   Before–after (i.e. repeated measures without control)
C   Before–after with control
D   Solomon four-group (special combination of A and C)
E   Other

Column heading: VP (video/programme conditions)
v   (intervention) video
p   (intervention) programme including video (e.g. video and discussion)
h   (comparison) video on another health topic
i   (comparison) video on a topic irrelevant to health
o   other intervention (no video)
n   no treatment/intervention.

All conditions are listed; e.g. vpon would refer to a design with four conditions, such as (v) video; (p) video and discussion; (o) leaflet; (n) no intervention control.

Column heading: FU (follow-up)
I   immediate
3 mn   3 months, etc.

AIDS and STDs

Study	Country	Theoretical perspective	Aim	DES	VP	FU	Sample Size	Group	Outcome
Adolescents and familes									
1. Balassone et al., 1993	USA	Reasoned action/SL	Develop 2 interventions for condom use	A	vo	–	89	Adolescents 16 years	1. Understood video 2. Would recommend to friends
2. Rickert et al., 1990	USA	Information	Compare 3 programmes	A	pon	–	75	Females, sexually active	1. Increase in knowledge for all groups 2. No change in attitude or condom use
3. Rickert et al., 1991	USA	Information	Compare peer-led v. adult-led programme	A	pon	–	82	Adolescents	1. More questions asked of peer, but both leaders equally effective in changing knowledge and attitude 2. Perceived susceptibility higher for those who viewed more 'affective' tape, particularly for those not sexually active
4. Slonim-Nevo et al., 1991	USA/ Israel	Information	Evaluate video	C	pn	– 1 mn	54	Youth from residential centre	No change in behaviour
5. Winett et al., 1992	USA	Social learning	Family-based programme to increase teens' skills, family problem-solving	C	vn	2 wks	45	Families	Increase in parent and teen knowledge after video
6. Winett et al., 1993	USA	Social learning	As above	C	pp	2 wks 4 mn	69	Families	Improved communication and knowledge after skill training video
High-risk groups									
7. Card et al., 1993	USA	Information	Assess multiple intervention	B	poo	3 mn	328	High-risk men, black	Increase in knowledge
8. Crawford and Robinson, 1990	USA	Information	Study knowledge	A	vvn	–	257	High-risk women, black	No increase in knowledge

AIDS and STDs
(continued)

Study	Country	Theoretical perspective	Aim	DES	VP	FU	Sample Size	Group	Outcome
9. Kalichman et al., 1993	USA	Information	Assess culturally sensitive package	B	vvv	2 wks	106	High-risk women, black	After all videos: 1. gains in knowledge; 2. more likely to discuss with friends, be tested for HIV and request condoms; 3. no effect on intention to practise safe sex
10. Maibach and Flora, 1993	USA	Social learning	Assess information + cognitive rehearsal on self-efficacy	B	vvv	1 mn	138	Unmarried women	Self-efficacy improved in video + rehearsal group
11. Meyer et al., 1992	USA	HBM	Assess programme	B	poo	3 mn	12	Mentally ill	1. Increase in knowledge 2. Improved attitude
12. Moizuddin, 1990	USA	Information	Assess programme	C	vn	1 mn	100	STD clinic patients	No effect on knowledge, but poor test (ceiling effects)
13. Perry et al., 1991	USA	Not stated	Compare 3 methods to reduce anxiety after screening for HIV	B	poo	3 mn	380	High-risk	1. For seronegative patients: decrease in distress for all 3 methods 2. For seropositive patients: awareness and self-reported condom use improved
14. Robert and Rosser, 1990	Australia	Social learning	Compare 5 programmes	C	vooon	6 mn	159	Homosexual men	1. No difference between programmes but ceiling effects, most practising safe sex before 2. Ceiling effects, most practising safe sex before
15. Singh and Malaviya, 1994	India	Information	Describes programme	B	p	2 yrs	811	Prostitutes	Awareness and self-reported condom use improved
16. Solomon and Dejong, 1988	USA	Social learning HBM	Improve clinic attendance	A	vn	2 wks	1153	STD clinic, black	Video produced better clinic attendance and knowledge
17. Solomon and Dejong, 1989	USA	Social learning	Assess effect of video + free condoms	A	vn	—	82	STD clinic, 80% black	Video group more likely to redeem coupons for condoms

Students, adults

Study	Country	Theoretical perspective	Aim	DES	VP	FU	Sample Size	Group	Outcome
18. Berrenberg et al., 1990–91	USA	Attribution	Determine impact of prevention programme on attitude to victims	A	vo	—	39	Undergrads 26 years	Video led to victim being denigrated, blamed for not preventing infection
19. Brown, 1991	USA	Communication	Assess effect of information on communication	C	vn	—	257	Undergrads inc. Asian	1. Increase in accurate beliefs and personal vulnerability 2. No effect on communication
20. Gilliam and Seltzer, 1989	USA	Information	Evaluate basic programme	C	vo	6 wks	278	Undergrads mostly black	1. Little effect on knowledge 2. Little effect on reported behaviour
21. Johnson et al., 1990	USA	Information	Assess educational programme	C	pn	2 mn	122	Medical students	1. Increase in knowledge 2. No effect on attitude
22. Kyes, 1990	USA	Personality	Assess video showing condom use	C	vvvi	—	160	Undergrads	1. Safe sex film led to more positive attitudes to condoms. 2. No effect on redeeming coupons for condoms
23. Lipson and Brown, 1991	USA	Information	Compare 3 videos on knowledge, attitude	C	vvvh	—	144	Undergrads	1. Increase in knowledge 2. Improved attitudes to people with AIDS
24. Muskin and Stevens, 1990	USA	Information 'affective'	Change prejudice toward AIDS patients	B	p	—	23	Medical students	Change in students' reported behaviour
25. Pryor et al., 1991	USA	Information TRA	Assess video to change attitudes to victims	A	vi	— 4–6 wk	250	Undergrads	More positive attitudes overall, no change among anti-homosexuals
26. Rhodes and Wolitski, 1989	USA	Information	Compare 4 videos	C	vvvvn	—	584	Undergrads	Increase in knowledge for 3 of 4 tapes
27. Sawyer and Beck, 1991	USA	HBM	Compare 2 videos on perceived susceptibility	C	vvnn	—	293	Undergrads	No effect on intention to perform safe sex

Alcohol

Study	Country	Theoretical perspective	Aim	DES	VP	FU	Sample Size	Group	Outcome
Adolescents									
1. Bochner, 1994	Australia	Social learning	Compare same- v. opposite-sex models	A	vvvv		95	16 yrs	1. Same-sex models more effective in reducing intention 2. Moderate drinkers more influenced than heavy
2. Collins and Cellucci, 1991	USA	Information	To assess an alcohol education presentation with a media component	C	PO	1 mn	52	Schools 16–17 yrs	1. Knowledge increased 2. No effect on attitudes and involvement
3. Duryea, 1983	USA	Inoculation	Compare package v. no treatment	D	po		155	14 yrs	Package associated with more knowledge, refuting arguments, compliance
4. Duryea et al., 1984	USA	Inoculation	Follow-up of study 3	D	po	6 mn	83	14 yrs	Knowledge and intentions still better than controls
5. Lignell and Hizar, 1991	USA	Information	To evaluate drug and alcohol education programme	B	p		180	School 14 yrs	Some changes in attitude
Patients									
6. Alterman and Baughman, 1991	USA	Information	To compare methods of giving information	B	ov	24 hrs	126	Alcoholics & outpatients	Gain in knowledge for all, no difference in amount gained
7. Baker et al., 1975	USA	Social learning	Evaluate video to train alcoholics to achieve controlled drinking	C	oppo	6 wks 6 mn	40	Alcoholics 25–55 yrs	1. All interventions better than standard treatment in producing controlled drinking 2. Self-confrontation video best
8. Craigie and Ross, 1980	USA	Social learning	Encourage detoxification patients to seek treatment	A	pp		31	Alcoholics	Modelling video + discussion better than exhortative video + discussion in getting patients to seek treatment

Alcohol

(continued)

Study	Country	Theoretical perspective	Aim	DES	VP	FU	Sample Size	Group	Outcome
9. Greer and Callis, 1975	USA	Social learning	Compare modelling with standard procedure	C	vo	30 dys	68	Alcoholics, male	Video led to less neuroticism, more self-confidence and willingness to take further treatment
10. McMurran and Lismore, 1993	UK	Social learning	To teach learning-disabled about alcohol problems	B	P?	?	2	Low IQ 44 and 35 yr	Subjects suggested more strategies
11. Stalonas et al., 1979	USA	Social learning	Evaluate self-management v. detoxification	B	opo	1 mn	48	Alcoholics	1. Increased knowledge in all groups, but most for total package 2. No difference between SL and detoxification
Adults									
12. Albert and Hodgson, 1984	Canada	Information Self-monitoring	To evaluate the impact of score card	C	PP	7–10 dy	108	Employees	1. Score card acceptable 2. No effect on attitudes or behaviour
13. Engs, 1977	USA	Information	To pilot campus-based awareness programme	C	VH	3 mn	83	Students	1. Knowledge improved 2. No effect on behaviour
14. McDermott et al., 1991	USA	Information	To assess method of training counsellors about alcohol problems	C	PO	3 wks	28	Counselling students M = 23 yrs	Effect on objective knowledge
15. Plant et al., 1979	UK	Information	To assess effect of TV-based campaign on knowledge and behaviour	A	VV	0–2 6–8	2516	General M = 46 yrs	1. Viewers: better knowledge 2. No effect on actual help-seeking 3. Viewers more likely to be drinkers
16. Strickler et al., 1981	USA	Social learning	To train drinkers to adopt controlled drinking style	C	VPPN	2 wks	32	Male college students, heavy social drinkers 19–24 yrs	1. Video only: no effect 2. Packages improved moderate drinking
17. Waterson and Murray-Lyon, 1990	UK	Information	To compare methods of advice	C	PO	28 wks after delivery	2100	Pregnant women	No effects

Drugs

Study	Country	Theoretical perspective	Aim	DES	VP	FU	Sample Size	Group	Outcome
1. Donohew et al., 1990	USA	Personality	Study individual differences in reactions to messages about marijuana	B	vvoo	I	342	High school	1. Video no better than print on attitude, intention, or acceptability 2. Arousal dependent on style, medium and sensation-seeking score
2. Eiser and Eiser, 1988 (study 1)	UK	Life skills	Assess use of video in school	A	p	8 mn	1000	Teachers	1. Video used widely, especially in health or PSME course 2. Teacher attitudes important in whether they chose package
3. Eiser and Eiser, 1988 (study 2)	UK	Life skills	Evaluate life-skills programme (A)	C	pn	2 wks	136	Schoolchildren 15–16 years	1. Video group evaluated drugs more negatively 2. Change to seeing drug use as situationally dependent rather than family background
4. Eiser and Eiser, 1988 (study 3)	UK	Life skills	Evaluate life-skills programme (B)	B	p	2 wks	124	Schoolchildren 14–15 years	More licit drugs regarded as addictive
5. Eiser and Eiser, 1988 (study 4)	UK	Life skills	Compare life-skills videos (A) & (B)	A	vvn	I	518	14–16 years	Dramatic video (A) led to 1. more negative attitudes to illicit drugs and 2. more attributions to situational pressure
6. Eiser and Eiser, 1988 (study 5)	UK	Life skills	Compare high v. low use of programme	B	p	8 mn	815	14–16 yrs	Pupils in high user schools rated more drugs as dangerous, more situational attributions
7. Hecht et al., 1993	USA	Life skills Social learning	Evaluate programme on resistance skills	C	pvoo	1 mn	465	High school	Weak effect on attitudes and self-reported drug use
8. Vogt, 1977	USA	Information	Evaluate programme	D	pn	3 wks	80	12 yrs	No post-test differences in attitude

Smoking

Adolescents

Study	Country	Theoretical perspective	Aim	DES	VP	FU	Sample Size	Group	Outcome
1. Banspach et al., 1989	USA	Life skills	Compare video v. teacher discussion on knowledge	C	von	—	237	10–12 years	Both groups showed improvement in distinguishing health messages
2. Botvin et al., 1990	USA	Life skills	Compare ways of training teachers in use of programme	C	von	3 yrs	5954	High school 12–14 years	No differences between teachers trained by video and workshop
3. Evans et al., 1981	USA	Inoculation Social learning	Compare full v. resistance v. physiological feedback	C	pn	3 yrs	1352	Schools 12–14 years	Claimed drop in smoking in all intervention groups (design problems)
4. Greer, 1989	USA	Information	Evaluate video	A	V	—	1226	High school 9–19	Increased knowledge of risk (no comparison group)
5. Hammes and Petersen, 1986	USA	Social learning Life skills	Evaluate video and relate to self-esteem	C	pn	3 wks	95	Schools 11 plus	Video group more able to resist social pressure
6. Hirschman and Leventhal, 1989	USA	Social learning	Evaluate video	C	vv	1 wk	315	High school 11–13 years	Group who saw social video less likely to smoke and more able to identify symptoms
7. Katz et al., 1989	USA	Social learning	Evaluate social skills video	C	vn	—	63	High school 12–14	Increase in refusal skills
8. O'Neill et al., 1983	USA	Social learning	Comparison of 2 videos	C	vi	— 1 mn	54	Smokers and non-smokers 13 years	Modelling video led to more attitude change than information video
9. Patterson, 1984	USA	None	Adapt adult programme for schools	B	po	— 3 mn	21	Smokers	Reduced consumption
10. Pfau et al., 1992	USA	Inoculation	Assess effectiveness of inoculation video	C	vn	10 wks 25 wks	1047	High school 13 years	1. Video helped lessen slippage from anti-smoking attitude 2. Most effect for low self-esteem subjects

Smoking
(Continued)

Study	Country	Theoretical perspective	Aim	DES	VP	FU	Sample Size	Group	Outcome
11. Pfau and Bockern, 1994	USA	Inoculation	Compare peer- and/or adult-led session + booster	C	vn	I 1 yr	1047	High school 13 years	Modest persistence of attitude change 1 year later
12. Schinke et al., 1986	USA	Life skills	Evaluate skills-based video v. conventional health education	C	pn	6 mn 1 yr 2 yrs	65	High school 11 years	1. Increase in knowledge 2. Less increase in smoking
13. Sussman et al., 1986	USA	Life skills	Compare adolescents' and adults' views	B	v	I	45 52	Adolescents Parents (not related)	1. Adolescents interested in decision-making, adults in peer /media influence 2. Some increase in knowledge
14. Sussman et al., 1989	USA	Social learning	Compare 2 videos about smokeless tobacco	B	vv	I	388	High school 16 years	Both videos increased concern and perceived risk
15. Telch et al., 1990	USA	Life skills Social learning	Compare effectiveness of social influence video with and without peer leader	C	vo	I 7 mn	814	High school 12 years	1. Video plus peer leader better than video only in reducing smoking onset 2. Some generalisation to alcohol
Adults									
16. Dyer, 1983	UK	Information Fear-arousal	Assess fear-arousing programme	A	vn	I	1800	BBC viewers	1. Heavy smokers avoided programme 2. Some intentions to cut down
17. Hall et al., 1983	USA	Behaviour therapy	Compare video and motivation v. aversive training	B	po	I 12 wks 26 wks	35	Smokers 51 years	Motivation group showed bigger reduction in smoking
18. Hallett and Sutton, 1988	UK	Information Pharmacological	Evaluate video v. nicotine gum	A	voh	3, 4 12 mn	1328	Worksite	Video less effective than gum
19. Lane and Bennison, 1985	USA	Social learning Decision-making	Evaluate cessation programme	B	p	3 mn	233	Smokers	1. 66% not smoking at 3 months FU 2. Importance of social support

Smoking
(Continued)

Study	Country	Theoretical perspective	Aim	DES	VP	FU	Sample Size	Group	Outcome
20. Lichtenstein and Hollis, 1992	USA	Stages of change	Assess compliance	A	po	1 yr	1380	Smokers	Video useful in facilitating other forms of intervention
21. Marston and Bettencourt, 1988	USA	Life skills Information	Evaluate self-help video	B	v	1 mn 12 mn	101	Smokers 48 years	40% abstinent after 3 months (motivated and no control group)
22. Pederson et al., 1979	USA	Hypnosis	Compare different forms of hypnotherapy	A	po	1, 3 6 mn	65	Smokers 41 years	Abstention twice as high in live hypnotherapy group compared with video or relaxation
23. Price et al., 1991	USA	HBM	Compare 2 videos	C	vn	2–3 wks pre-delivery	193	Pregnant women (22 yrs)	No differences in quitting between videos and control group
24. Reeves et al., 1991	USA	Emotions	Compare effect of positive and negative emotions	A	vv	—	24	Undergrads 19–40 yrs	Attention better for positive messages
25. Schwarz et al., 1985	Germany	Information Attribution	To see if attributions mediate fear-arousal	C	vn	2 wks	49	Smokers, undergrads	1. Fear-arousal message can persuade 2. Watching video increased fear
26. Stevens et al., 1993	USA	Stages of change	Evaluate in-hospital intervention	C	pn	3 mn 12 mn	1119	Smokers 43 years	Abstinence higher than no intervention group
27. Sutton and Eiser, 1984	UK	SEU	Test fear-arousal	C	vn	3 mn	61	Smokers 35 years	1. Film affected fear and attempts to quit 2. Intention predicted behaviour and was predicted by confidence
28. Watson et al., 1983	UK	Fear-arousal	Compare arousal in response to fear message in smokers and non-smokers	B	v	—	20	Female 19–60	Film increased smokers' but not non-smokers' heart rate

Nutrition

Study	Country	Theoretical perspective	Aim	DES	VP	FU	Sample Size	Group	Outcome
1. Cotugna and Vickery, 1992	USA	Information	Evaluate videos on role of nutrition in reducing cancer risk	A	v	I	1050	Supermarket customers	No real evaluation; videos acceptable
2. Dougherty et al., 1990	USA	Information	Evaluate video in attitude to low fat foods	B	ppo	1 wk 6 mn	500	Shoppers	1. No increase in knowledge 2. No influence on sales
3. Greene and Strychar, 1992	USA	Health Belief	Improve diet after worksite cholesterol screening	C	vo	2 wks 4 mn	396	Employers	1. Improved knowledge and lower fat intake in participants 2. Participants more concerned about cholesterol 3. Best for lower educational levels
4. Lackey et al., 1992	USA	None	Compare video with personal assessment following cholesterol screening	A	vo	6 wks	382	Employers	No differences between groups on dietary change
5. Moreno and Thelen, 1993	USA	Information	Compare 2 videos	C	pn	2 dys 1 mn	167	Girls 13-14 yrs	Improved with regard to intent to diet, control weight
6. Pace et al., 1983	USA	Information	Evaluate video	C	vpn	1 wk 2 mn	68	Men 35-59 years with high cholesterol	1. Improved breakfast diet 2. Non-significant at 2-month follow-up 3. No change in knowledge or attitude
7. Peterson et al., 1984	USA	Hierarchy of effects	Evaluate TV programmes	C	vn	I	106	Children 5-6 years	Improved knowledge, attitude and behaviour for both intervention and control groups
8. Winett et al., 1988	USA	Social learning	Compare video, leaflet, lecture, modelling	C	6pn	7 wks	126	Shoppers 18-64	1. Most interventions better than controls 2. Interventions with modelling and feedback most effective in changing food purchase
9. Winett et al., 1991a	USA	Social learning	Evaluate interactive video	C	vn	2-8 wks	42	Shoppers 23-86	Increased purchase of high fibre foods
10. Winett et al., 1991b	USA	Social learning	Evaluate interactive video	C	vn	7-8 wks	69	Shoppers	Replicates study 9

Miscellaneous health promotion and prevention

Study	Country	Theoretical perspective	Aim	DES	VP	FU	Sample Size	Group	Outcome
Children and adolescents									
1. Carroll-Rowan and Miltenberger, 1994	USA	Social learning	Promote awareness of abduction	A	von	1 wk	62	4–5 yrs	Both interventions better than control (objective behavioural test)
2. Locketz, 1976	Surinam	Information	Develop programme for use in rural schools on infection control	B	v	–	?	Children 12 yrs	Qualitative interviews before and after suggest video acceptable and instructive
3. Meagher and Mann, 1990	Canada	Social learning	Compare video and leaflet on knowledge and attitude to blood pressure	B	pn	1 wk 3 mn	539	Adolescents 12–15 yrs	Video increased knowledge at 1 week but no differences at 3 months
4. Poche et al., 1988	USA	Information	Promote awareness of abduction	A	pvo	1 dy 1 mn	75	5–7 yrs	Package better than video alone (objective behavioural test)
5. Sarason et al., 1992	USA	Social learning	Compare video v. standard appeal to promote blood donation	A	vo	–	4970	High school 16–18 yrs	Video associated with more positive attitudes, intention and more donation
6. Sigurdson et al., 1987	Canada	Information	Promote awareness of sexual assault	B	vvvv	–	137	9–13 yrs	1. Video liked 2. Gain in knowledge and assertiveness significant for girls only
Adults									
Cody and Lee , 1990	Australia	HBM	Compare informational and emotional video in changing knowledge, behaviour and beliefs re skin cancer	C	vvh	– 10 wks	312	Undergrads	1. Both videos improved intentions 2. Effects of emotional video lasted longer
8. Hurtado and Hovell, 1993	USA	SL/decision-making	Compare various health videos	C	6v	–	299	Navy personnel	Back injury video associated with increased knowledge, no other effects

Miscellaneous health promotion and prevention

(Continued)

Study	Country	Theoretical perspective	Aim	DES	VP	FU	Sample Size	Group	Outcome
9. Miller et al., 1990	USA	Optimistic bias	Change stereotype of attractiveness of tan	B	vv	I	355	Undergrads	Video effective
10. Rossi et al., 1994	USA	None	Compare 9 interventions on sunbathing	E	vv7o	I	633	Beachgoers	Only reports agreement to participate
11. Sutton and Eiser, 1990	UK	Decision-making	Evaluate effects of fear-arousal	C	vv	I 3 mn	157	Clerical	Intention to wear seat belts mediated by film and fear-arousal
12. Sutton and Hallett, 1989	UK	Decision-making	Evaluate effects of fear-arousal	C	vh	I 3 mn 1 yr	227	Employees	Video influenced risk beliefs, fear and intention, fear important mediator of video effect on intention

Preparation for surgery

Study	Country	Theoretical perspective	Aim	DES	VP	FU	Sample Size	Group	Outcome
Children									
1. Bradlyn et al., 1986	USA	Social learning	To evaluate video to increase cooperation	C	voh	24 hrs	24	Cardiac catheterisation 4–16 years	No effect on behaviour or in reducing anxiety
2. Durst, 1990	USA	Coping	To evaluate video to reduce stress preoperatively	A	vv	—	59	Minor surgery 2–10 years	No effects on behaviour
3. Elkins and Roberts, 1985	USA	Social learning	To compare 3 videos: knowledge, attitude and behaviour, as function of self-efficacy	C	vvvi	— 3 wks	80	Healthy 8–11 years	1. High fear children showed less fear after any of 3 videos 2. No effects for low fear children 3. Effects of tape mediated by self-efficacy
4. Melamed et al., 1976	USA	Social learning	Evaluate timing of video	B	vv	— 5 wks	48	Elective surgery 4–12 years	1. Reduced anxiety 2. Younger children benefit more from immediate (v. delayed) view
5. Melamed and Siegel, 1975	USA	Social learning	Evaluate video	C	pi	— 3 wks	60	Minor surgery 4–12 years	1. Reduced anxiety 2. Fewer behaviour problems on discharge
6. Pinto and Hollandsworth, 1989	USA	Social learning	1. Compare parent presence/absence 2. Compare adult- v. peer-narrated tape	C	vvn	—	60	Minor surgery 2–12 years	1. Both videos associated with reduced anxiety and improved recovery 2. Those who viewed with parents were less distressed
7. Rasnake and Linscheid, 1989	USA	Cognitive developmental	To consider age differences in design of video	A	vvi	—	48	Gastroenterology 3–5 and 7–10 years	Video matched to developmental level associated with less distress but no effect on pulse rate or nurse rating

Preparation for surgery
(Continued)

Study	Country	Theoretical perspective	Aim	DES	VP	FU	Sample Size	Group	Outcome
8. Robinson and Kobayashi, 1991	Australia	Social learning	Compare modelling with child and parent coping skills	B	vvp	–	28	Minor surgery 4–13 years	No effects of training skills over modelling video
9. Twardosz et al., 1986	USA	Information	Compare video, class and nurse preparation	C	voo	–	60	Minor surgery 3–12 years	1. No differences on physiological measures 2. 'Class' associated with better behaviour than video 3. Worse behaviour for 'nurse' group
10. Uzark et al., 1982	USA	Information	Evaluate relevant v. irrelevant video	C	vi	– 4 wks	53	Cardiac catheterisation 3–12 years	1. Video associated with more knowledge, less disruptive behaviour and more questions asked 2. No differences in sleep disturbance
11. Peterson et al., 1984	USA	Social learning	Compare 3 methods: puppets, video, commercial film	C	vvv	–	44	Minor surgery 2–11 years	1. All 3 groups better than standard procedure (less anxiety) 2. No differences between interventions suggesting modelling important but not presentation
12. Ferguson, 1979	USA	Social learning	Compare modelling v. nurse pre-admission visit v. control	C	von	– 7 dys	82	Minor surgery 3–7 yrs	1. Previsit associated with less maternal anxiety and fewer post-hospital behaviour problems 2. Video associated with decrease in physiological arousal and better post-hospital behaviour

Preparation for surgery
(Continued)

Study	Country	Theoretical perspective	Aim	DES	VP	FU	Sample Size	Group	Outcome
Adults									
13. Gaskey, 1987	USA	Information	To evaluate video	C	vo	— 72 hrs	40	Gynaecology 33 years	1. Fewer symptoms in video group 2. Better knowledge 3. No effect on anxiety
14. Herrman and Kreuzer, 1989	Germany	Information	To evaluate video	C	po	—	65	Coronary angiography 58 years	1. Reduced anxiety 2. No effect on expectations about complications
15. Hill et al., 1988	USA	Information	Compare videos with nurse interview	C	vpo	—	30	Cardiac catheterisation 35–78 years	1. No differences in anxiety, knowledge or cooperation 2. Video is adjunct to personal contact
16. Mahler et al., 1993	USA	Social learning	To compare 3 videos to reduce anxiety	A	vvn	—	127	Undergrads (simulated) 16–25 years	1. Few differences between 3 videos; all reported less anxiety and more self-efficacy 2. 'Mastery' tape associated with less anxiety than 'coping'
17. Shipley et al., 1978	USA	Behavioural	Evaluate video	C	vv	—	60	Gastro clinic 22–80 years	Reduction in fear associated with video
18. Wicklin and Forster, 1994	USA	Social learning	Test whether personal video more helpful in reducing anxiety than information video	A	vvn	—	91	18–75 yrs outpatients	No effects
19. Hawkins and Price, 1993	Australia	Information	To encourage patients to ask for analgesia	C	pvo	48 hrs	60	Post-op 20–70 years	1. No differences between groups 2. 'Sensitisers' need different video
20. Holden et al., 1992	USA	Social learning	Compare structured v. unstructured setting	C	vv	—	93	Outpatients 50 yrs	Poor response to structured setting

Dentistry

Study	Country	Theoretical perspective	Aim	DES	VP	FU	Sample Size	Group	Outcome
Children									
1. Fields and Pinkham, 1976	USA	Social learning	Compare modelling video with pretreatment visit or none	C	vvn	I	24	Children (3–5 years) (first appointment)	No behaviour differences between 3 groups
2. Del Gaudio and Nevid, 1991	USA	Social learning	1. Assess effect of coping skills training 2. Compare dental v. classroom setting	C	ppvo oo	2 wks	68	Anxious children (9–13 yrs)	1. Multicomponent treatment most effective for anxiety 2. No effect for behaviour or physiological measures
3. Zachary et al.,1985	USA	Social learning	Effects of stress-relevant v. irrelevant information on coping	C	vhi	I	53	Children (3–11 yrs)	No difference between relevant and irrelevant information
4. Rouleau et al., 1981	Canada	Social learning	Compare live or video	A	vvvi	24 hrs	38	Children (4–6 years)	1. No differences between video groups 2. Little anxiety on first visit
5. Klingman et al., 1984	USA	Social learning	Compare modelling with active coping information	C	pv	I	38	Fearful children (8–13 years)	More use of active coping compared with modelling
6. McMurray et al., 1985	Australia	Social learning	Compare modelling and mastery tapes on anxiety and behaviour	C	vvh	I	24	Fearful children (5–7 years)	Both videos more effective than placebo
7. Melamed et al., 1978	USA	Social learning	Compare modelling and information	C	vovoi	I	80	Dental patients (4–11 years)	1. Modelling better than information 2. Effect depends on age, experience

Dentistry
(Continued)

Study	Country	Theoretical perspective	Aim	DES	VP	FU	Sample Size	Group	Outcome
Adults									
8. Auerbach et al., 1976	USA	Social learning	1. Compare general v. specific videos in reducing anxiety 2. Mediating effect of locus of control	B	vi	I post-surgery	63	Dental patients (19–74 yrs)	1. 'Internals' viewing specific compared with general video less anxious 2. No simple evaluation of general v. specific videos
9. Davis et al., 1986	USA	Information	Evaluate information video in terms of expectations and satisfaction	C	vi	I 6 wks	81	Dental patients (40–81 yrs)	1. No effect of video on expectations about dentures 2. Modelling group showed some advantage when controlling for anxiety
10. Gatchel, 1986	USA	Coping/ desensitisation	Evaluate coping skills video on reducing fear	C	vi	I 6 mn	40	Public (over 21 yrs)	1. Moderately fearful more likely to make appointment 2. No effect on very fearful
11. Kois et al., 1978	USA	None described	Compare personal supervision v. video in teaching plaque removal	C	ppp	I	42 42	Technicians Patients	1. No difference between interventions 2. No effect on behaviour 3. No difference between groups
12. Moore et al., 1991	Denmark	Desensitisation	Assess video/clinic rehearsal on anxiety reduction	C	pon	I 1 yr	143	Dental fear patients	1. Interventions did not differ 2. Both led to reduced fear 3. Most consulted dentist within 1 year
13. Robertson et al., 1991	USA	Coping	Compare behavioural therapy video with placebo video and no treatment	C	phn	I	60	Patients	1. Treatment video rated most 2. Treatment resulted in reduced arousal 3. No effect on behaviour

Screening

Study	Country	Theoretical perspective	Aim	DES	VP	FU	Sample Size	Group	Outcome
1. Banks et al., 1995	USA	Prospect	Compare effectiveness of loss-framed v. gain-framed information in mammography screening	B	vv 6 mn 12 mn	l	133	Population 40–60 years	Women more likely to attend if given loss-framed information
2. Ehmann, 1993	USA	Information	Promote breast awareness	A	p	nil	109	High school	Video acceptable
3. Fisher et al., 1981	USA	Information	Compare video v. live counselling after screening	C	vo	l	96	Adults 37 yrs	1. Knowledge increased for both groups 2. Videos save professional time
4. Hill and Gardner, 1980	Australia	Personality	Determine differences between repressors and sensitisers in reacting to threat video	A	vvv	l 6 wks	79	Males 23–63	1. Intention to attend screening higher for sensitisers 2. High threat more effective for repressors
5. McAvoy and Raza, 1991	UK	Information	Compare 3 methods in influencing women to take up smear test	A	oopn	2 wks 4 mn	737	Asian women 18-52	Uptake good following video or personal visit compared with leaflet alone
6. O'Brien and Lee, 1990	Australia	HBM	Assess effect of modelling on uptake of screening	C	vv	l 5 wks	245	Women 16–63	1. Increase in knowledge and risk factors after film 2. Strong effect on behaviour
7. Ser Vaas and Weinberger, 1979	USA	None	Compare motivation pack for hypertension screening with standard advice	E	o	6 wks	477	Adults	78% package group and 28% standard group sought appropriate follow-up

Patient education

Study	Country	Theoretical perspective	Aim	DES	VP	FU	Sample Size	Group	Outcome
Asthma									
1. Holzheimer et al., 1995	Australia	Social learning	Compare video and leaflets	C	pooi	— 1 mn	80	Asthma 2–5yrs	All showed increased knowledge and management compared with controls; video and leaflet best
2. Moldofsky et al., 1979	Canada	Information	Increase knowledge Assess relationship between knowledge and medical status	C	vn	— 16 mn	79	Adults with asthma no effect on medical status	Increased knowledge after video, no difference at follow-up, no effect on medical status
3. Partridge, 1986	UK	Information	Compare video and leaflets	A	v	—	66	Asthma 5–75 yrs	No real evaluation
Renal disease									
4. Barbour and Blumenkrantz, 1978	USA	Information	Achieve informed consent	B	vn	—	132	Dialysis patients	Increase in number giving informed consent
5. Lawson et al., 1976	USA	Information	Increase dietary compliance	C	vo	— 1 mn	30	Dialysis patients	1. Increase in knowledge 2. Improved self-reported compliance
Diabetes									
6. Bethea et al., 1989	USA	Not given	Compare video with conventional instruction	B	ov	—	24	Adults with diabetes	No differences between interventions
7. Brown et al., 1992	Mexico	Information	Effect of video on increasing knowledge	C	vv	—	30	Adults	Increase in knowledge and acceptability of media
8. Gilbert et al., 1982	USA	Social learning	Effect of peer modelling on anxiety reduction and skill acquisition	C	po	— 4 dys	28	Children 6–9 yrs	1. No effect on anxiety 2. Improved self-injection for older girls

Patient education
(Continued)

Study	Country	Theoretical perspective	Aim	DES	VP	FU	Sample Size	Group	Outcome
9. McCulloch et al., 1983	UK	Information	Compare 3 interventions on compliance, knowledge and metabolic control	C	opp	6 mn	40	Adults with diabetes	1. Improvement for all intervention groups 2. Compliance intervention most effective
10. McCulloch et al., 1985	UK	Information	Compare demonstration v. video	C	po	6 mn	40	Diabetes 17–64 yrs	Both groups more knowledgeable, compliant and better metabolic control than control group
11. Pichert et al., 1994	USA	Social learning	Instruct adolescents about sick day management	C	po	2 wks	81	Adolescents with diabetes	No effect on knowledge
Cardiac conditions									
12. Bracken et al., 1977	USA	None	Compare video v. lecture in increasing knowledge	C	vo	I	45	Cardiac patients M = 55 yrs	1. No difference for young patients 2. Older knew more, following video
13. Brandao et al., 1992	USA	Information	Compare dietitian, classroom, slide and video on knowledge	A	vopn	I	153	Coronary patients and spouse 30–80 years	Increase in knowledge for all intervention groups; no difference between interventions
Miscellaneous									
14. Anderson et al., 1987	USA	Social learning	Compare 2 videos (modelling v. information)	C	vvv	I	150	Male 27–76	Modelling video better in improving communication (but not if subject's motivation controlled for)
15. Barry and Daniels, 1984	USA	Information	Reduce missed appointments	A	von	11 mn	317	Outpatients	Improved attendance for video group compared with leaflet or no information

Patient education
(Continued)

Study	Country	Theoretical perspective	Aim	DES	VP	FU	Sample Size	Group	Outcome
16. Buckley et al., 1981	USA	Information	Compare video v. practice in teaching home monitoring	A	vo	1 wk	20	Hypertensives 13–18 yrs	Both methods equally effective
17. Hamilton et al., 1993	USA	HBM	Compare standard care with package to improve adherence	C	po	6 mn	34	Hypertensives 54 yrs	Package associated with improved appointment-keeping
18. Koperski, 1989	UK	None	Assess acceptability of video in waiting room	A	v		161	Patients	Videos acceptable, no evaluation of knowledge or attitude
19. McGowan et al., 1994	USA	Behaviour modification	Compare nutrition/ behaviour programme with lecture and video	C	po	8 wks 8 mn	39	Undergraduates with high B 18 years	Improved knowledge and cholesterol levels in video group compared with controls
20. Rosenthal et al., 1983	USA UK	Information	Educate patients about ophthalmology	C	v	6 mn	162	Glaucoma patients and controls	Improvement in knowledge
21. Sanguinetti and Catanzaro, 1987	USA	Information	Prepare family to care for patient with brain injury	A	po		29	Families of patients	Improved knowledge and skills to handle problems
22. Stone et al., 1989	USA	Information	Compare video and lecture	C	vo		22	Patients 59 yrs	No differences in knowledge

Parenting

Pregnancy and labour

Study	Country	Theoretical perspective	Aim	DES	VP	FU	Sample Size	Group	Outcome
1. Bachman et al., 1992	USA	Information	Educate parents about symptoms of premature labour	A	v	I	418	Women	1. No formal measure of knowledge 2. Women liked video and reported understanding
2. Cobiella et al., 1990	USA	Coping skills	Devise parent coping stategies	C	vvv	I	30	Mothers with high-risk infant in NICU	1. Reduced anxiety for problem-focused group 2. Lower depression for emotion group
3. Daelhousen and Guthrie, 1982	USA	Information HBM	Assess effectiveness of nutrition programme	C	pn	I	52	Pregnant women 24 yrs	1. Improved knowledge 2. No change in attitude or behaviour
4. Freda et al., 1990	USA	Information	Educate women about dangers of prematurity and signs of premature labour	C	p	I	615	Women high-risk	Increase in knowledge but video part of intervention package
5. Freda et al., 1988	USA	TRA	Increase awareness of problems of pre-term birth	C	vo	I 1 mn	66	Professional staff 21–68 yrs	Awareness of problems of premature birth and reported intentions to change behaviour
6. Manderino and Bzdek, 1984	USA	Information Social learning	Reduce pain during labour	A	vvvi	I	60	Female students (simulated situation)	Those who saw video reported less pain than irrelevant video, but not clear if relevant to real situation
7. Mynaugh, 1991	USA	Information	Compare 2 methods of teaching perineal massage	C	pv	I	83	Pregnant	No effects on delivery experience

Parenting
(Continued)

Parent education

Study	Country	Theoretical perspective	Aim	DES	VP	FU	Sample Size	Group	Outcome
8. Kleemeier and Hazzard, 1984	USA	Information	Compare video on parenting tips in structured v. unstructured setting	A	vv	–	120	Parents 26 years	Increase in knowledge more in structured setting
9. Koniak-Griffin et al., 1992	USA	Social learning	Improve mothering skills	C	po 2 mn	–	31	Adolescent mothers	Improved attitude and mothering skills
10. Paperny, 1992	USA	None	Assess value of video to enhance advice	E	p	–	204	Parents	Videos rated helpful but no real evaluation
11. Rossiter, 1994	Australia	TPB	Promote breast feeding	C	pn	–	266	Pregnant Vietnamese	Increased knowledge and breast feeding at 4 weeks, not sustained by 6 months

Studies involving social learning models

1. Health promotion and prevention

Study	Comparison	Results	Comments
AIDS (*n* = 27)			
5	(i) Video plus practice (ii) None	Increase in knowledge and skills for video group	
6	(i) Video plus information and skills training (ii) Video with information only	(i) Both resulted in increased knowledge (ii) Skills training associated with improved communication	
10	(i) Information video (ii) Information plus modelling video (iii) Above plus cognitive rehearsal	(i) Self-efficacy most improved for information plus model plus rehearsal group (ii) Information plus modelling intermediate	
14	(i) Information video (ii) Individual counselling (iii) Group programme (iv) Group programme (v) No intervention	No differences between interventions	Most already practising safe sex
15	(i) Video (ii) No intervention	Experimental group better in appointments, also better knowledge	
Alcohol (*n* = 17)			
1	(i) Discussion of drinking by same-sex model (ii) Same discussion by other-sex model	(i) 'Matched' message led to higher evaluation of speaker and message (ii) Lighter drinkers evaluated more positively	
3	(i) Video plus role play (ii) Nothing	Intervention group better in knowledge, attitude and refuting arguments and reported compliance	
4	As above	Difference maintained at 6-month FU	
7	(i) Behaviour counselling (ii) Counselling plus video (self) (iii) Counselling plus model controlled drinking (iv) Standard treatment	(i) All interventions better than control (ii) Self-confrontation best (iii) Modelling less effective than counselling alone	
8	(i) Video plus specific discussion (ii) Video plus general discussion	Experimental group more likely to accept referral for treatment	
9	(i) Video plus discussion (ii) Standard procedure	Experimental group less neurotic, more self-confident and agree to treatment	
10	(i) Video showing drink problems (ii) Nothing	Video better	

Study	Comparison	Results	Comments
11	(i) Live (ii) Video of above (iii) Above by social learn programme (iv) Above by detoxification	(i) All groups improved in knowledge, strongest for video (ii) No difference between SL and detoxification	
16	(i) Rationale video (ii) Plus self-monitoring form (iii) Plus practice video	Moderate drinking improved in both self-monitoring and practice conditions especially practice	

Drugs (*n* = 8)

5 of 8 articles based on SL but not so that appropriate comparisons can be made

Smoking (*n* = 28)

Study	Comparison	Results	Comments
1	(i) Video resisting social pressures (ii) Teacher-led discussion (iii) No intervention	Both interventions better than control in identifying messages in adverts	
2	(i) Teachers trained by workshop (ii) Trained by video	Intervention groups better in smoking and marijuana	
3	(i) Full treatment (ii) Resist pressure group (iii) Physio feedback (iv) No intervention	Poor analysis	
5	(i) Intervention (ii) None	Suggests resistance to persuasion can be taught	
6	(i) Skills training (ii) Information videos	Experimental group better than video in terms of not taking 2nd cigarette	
7	(i) Video (ii) No intervention	Video better in refusal skills	
8	(i) Video on negative consequences of smoking (ii) Video on reasons for smoking	Experimental group better attitudes	
10	(i) Video peer-led (ii) Video adult-led (iii) Both (iv) Nothing	Positive results only for those with poor self-esteem	
11	As above	Modest persistence of attitude change later	
12	(i) Video with skills intervention (ii) Video with conventional message	Less increase in smoking for skills group	
13		Not evaluative	
14	4 videos 2 x 2 emotions x probability	(i) Emotions had no effect (ii) High probability video most successful	

Study	Comparison	Results	Comments
15	(i) Video plus peer leader (ii) Video only (iii) Survey	Video and peer leader better than video alone in inhibiting smoking	
19	(i) 6 interventions involving everything (ii) Nothing	Those who attended all less likely to smoke	
21	Video no control	Good proportion abstinent at follow-up	

Nutrition _n_ = 8

Study	Comparison	Results	Comments
7	Video, leaflets, lecture, modelling	Modelling plus feedback	

Miscellaneous health promotion/prevention

Study	Comparison	Results	Comments
1	(i) Video plus rehearsal (ii) Teacher taught (iii) No training control	(i) Rehearsal and teacher groups better than no training control in self-report and behaviour (ii) 0% teacher group, 9% video group and 22% controls went with stranger	
3	(i) Video and discussion (ii) Completed questionnaire	At 1 wk, video group more knowledgeable, this gone at 3 months	
5	(i) Video (ii) Standard appeal	(i) Video led to more positive attitude and intention to donate blood (ii) Donation higher in video group	

2. Healthcare settings

Study	Comparison	Results	Comments

Surgery (_n_ = 20)

Study	Comparison	Results	Comments
1	(i) Modelling video (ii) Standard information plus tour (iii) Information video	No differences between groups	(i) Experienced group (ii) Big age range (4–16)
3	(i) Modelling video (ii) Information video (iii) Slide and audiotape (iv) Irrelevant video	(i) High-fear children showed reduced fear after all interventions (ii) No difference between interventions	
4	(i) Modelling video day before admission (ii) Same 9 days before admission	Reduction in anxiety and improved behaviour following video	Greater effectiveness of model when seen to be similar
5	(i) Modelling video plus standard care (ii) Standard admission policy	Modelling group showed reduced anxiety etc. compared with standard admission group	

Study	Comparison	Results	Comments
6	(i) Adult-narrated video (ii) Peer-narrated video	No differences between videos or depending on parent presence	
8	(i) Modelling video (information) (ii) Modelling video (child coping) (iii) Modelling video (child and parent coping skills)	(i) No differences between 3 groups (ii) Attributed to previous experience	
11	(i) Information puppet show (ii) Modelling video (iii) Modelling video	(i) All interventions better than control group (ii) No differences between modelling groups	

Adults

Study	Comparison	Results	Comments
12	(i) Modelling video plus pre-admission visit (ii) Visit only	Intervention group reported fewer symptoms and more knowledgeable	
16	(i) Nurse gives information (ii) Mastery video (iii) Coping video	(i) Both videos assoc with less anxiety and more self-efficacy than nurse group (ii) Mastery group least anxious	Effect of tapes may be mediated by self-efficacy beliefs
18	(i) Personally relevant video (ii) Information (iii) No video	(i) No effects of either video (ii) No differences between 3 groups	

Dentistry *n* = 13

Study	Comparison	Results	Comments
1	(i) Modelling video (ii) Pre-treatment visit (iii) Nothing	No behaviour differences for 3 groups	Low anxiety and disruptive behaviour
2	(i) Multicomponent plus modelling video (ii) As above without video (iii) Modelling video only (iv) Coping skills training (v) Discussion group (vi) Waiting list control	(i) Most effective in reducing anxiety (ii) No effects on behaviour or physiological function	
3	(i) Modelling video (ii) Irrelevant video (iii) Neutral film	No differences on behaviour or attitude	Inappropriate model
4	(i) One showing of video (ii) Two showings of video (iii) Live presentation of same (iv) Placebo control	No effect on behaviour	Little initial anxiety
5	(i) Modelling video plus rehearsal (ii) Modelling video only	Rehearsal group showed more positive coping	
6	(i) Mastery video (ii) Coping video (iii) Placebo tape	(i) Mastery and coping videos showed reduction in anxiety compared with placebo (ii) No difference between mastery and coping (iii) No differences between 3 groups on behaviour	

Study	Comparison	Results	Comments
7	(i) Long modelling video (ii) Long demonstration (iii) Short modelling video (iv) Short demonstration (v) Unrelated film	(i) Modelling video superior to demonstrations	Importance of age and previous experience

Adults

None used SL

Screening (*n* = 7)

None used SL

Patient education (*n* = 22)

1	(i) Video and book (ii) Video and unrelated book (iii) Unrelated video and asthma book (iv) Unrelated video and book	(i) All intervention groups increased in knowledge (ii) Video and related book best (iii) Better management by all intervention groups	
8	(i) Modelling video (ii) Diet video	(i) No difference in anxiety between groups (ii) Modelling video better for older girls	
11	(i) Video on problem-solving (ii) Small group teaching session	(i) No difference on knowledge (ii) Intervention group better at explanations	
14	(i) Modelling video (ii) Same information but no model	Modelling video associated with more question-asking	

Parenting (*n* = 11)

4	(i) Modelling video (ii) Information video (iii) Modelling and information video	Combined video and information more successful than either alone in terms of reported pain	Subjects were students, relevance to real pain unclear
11	(i) Videotaped own behaviour plus rehearsal and feedback (ii) Video only, no rehearsal	Videoed instruction and feedback resulted in better mothering than video only	

References

AIDS and STDs

Adolescents and families

1. Balassone, M. L., Baker, S., Gillmore, M. R., Morrison, D., and Dickstein, D. (1993). Interventions to decrease the risk of HIV/AIDS and other sexually transmitted diseases among high-risk heterosexual adolescents. *Children and Youth Services Review*, **15**, 475–88.

2. Rickert, V. I., Gottlieb, A., and Jay, M. S. (1990). A comparison of three clinic-based AIDS education programs on female adolescents' knowledge, attitudes, and behavior. *Journal of Adolescent Health Care*, **11**, 298–303.

3. Rickert, V. I., Jay, M. S., and Gottlieb, A. (1991). Effects of a peer-counseled AIDS education program on knowledge, attitudes, and satisfaction of adolescents. *Journal of Adolescent Health*, **12**, 38–43.

4. Slonim-Nevo, V., Ozawa, M. N., and Auslander, W. F. (1991). Knowledge, attitudes and behaviors related to AIDS among youth in residential centers: results from exploratory study. *Journal of Adolescence*, **14**, 17–33.

5. Winett, R. A., Anderson, E. S., Moore, J. F., Sikkema, K. J., Taylor, C. D., Hook, R. J., Webster, D. A., Dalton, J. E., Ollendick, T. H. and Eisler, R. M. (1992). Family/media approach to HIV prevention: results with a home-based, parent-teen video program. *Health Psychology*, **11**, 203–6.

6. Winett, R. A., Anderson, E. S., Moore, J. F., Taylor, C. D., Hook, R. J., Webster, D. A., Neubauer, T. E., Harden, M. C., and Mundy, L. L. (1993). Efficacy of home-based human immunodeficiency virus prevention video program for teens and parents. *Health Education Quarterly*, **20**, 555–67.

High-risk groups

7. Card, C. A. L., Jacobsberg, L. B., Moffatt, M., Fishman, B., and Perry, S. (1993). Using interactive video to supplement HIV counseling. *Hospital and Community Psychiatry*, **44**, 383–5.

8. Crawford, I. and Robinson, W. L. (1990). Adolescents and AIDS: knowledge and attitudes of African-American, Latino, and Caucasian Midwestern US high school seniors. *Journal of Psychology and Human Sexuality*, **3**, 25–33.

9. Kalichman, S. C., Kelly, J. A., Hunter, T. L., Murphy, D. A., and Tyler, R. (1993). Culturally-tailored HIV-AIDS risk-reduction messages targeted to African-American urban women: impact on risk sensitization and risk reduction. *Journal of Consulting and Clinical Psychology*, **61**, 291–5.

10. Maibach, E. and Flora, J. A. (1993). Symbolic modeling and cognitive rehearsal: using video to promote AIDS prevention self-efficacy. *Communication Research*, **20**, 517–45.

11. Meyer, I., Cournos, F., Empfield, M., Agosin, B., and Floyd, P. (1992). HIV prevention among psychiatric inpatients: a pilot risk reduction study. *Psychiatric Quarterly*, **63**, 187–97.

12. Moizuddin, S. P. (1990). Impact of clinic based educational videotape on knowledge of AIDS in STD patients. *Journal of the Florida Medical Association*, **77**, 40–2.

13. Perry, S., Fishman, B., Jacobsberg, L., Young, J., and Frances, A. (1991). Effectiveness of psychoeducational interventions in reducing emotional distress after human immunodeficiency virus antibody testing. *Archives of General Psychiatry*, **48**, 143–7.

14. Robert, B. and Rosser, S. (1990). Evaluation of the efficacy of AIDS education interventions for homosexually active men. *Health Education Research: Theory and Practice*, **5**, 299–308.

15. Singh, Y. N. and Malaviya, N. M. (1994). Experience of HIV prevention interventions among female sex workers in Delhi, India. *International Journal of STD & AIDS*, **5**, 56–7.

16. Solomon, M. Z. and DeJong, W. (1988). The impact of a clinic-based educational videotape on knowledge and treatment behavior of men with gonorrhea. *Sexually Transmitted Diseases*, **15**, 127–32.

17. Solomon, M. Z. and DeJong, W. (1989). Preventing AIDS and other STDs through condom promotion: a patient education intervention. *American Journal of Public Health*, **79**, 453–8.

Students/adults

18. Berrenberg, J. L., Rosnik, D., and Kravcisin, N. J. (1990-91). Blaming the victim: when disease-prevention programs misfire. *Current Psychology: Research and Reviews*, **9**, 415–20.

19. Brown, W. J. (1991). An AIDS prevention campaign: effects on attitudes, beliefs, and communication behavior. *American Behavioral Scientist*, **34**, 666–78.

20. Gilliam, A. and Seltzer, R. (1989) The efficacy of educational movies on AIDS knowledge and attitudes among college students. *Journal of American College Health*, **37**, 261–5.

21. Johnson, J. A., Campbell, A. E., Toewe, C. H. and Bell, B. J. (1990). Knowledge and attitudes about AIDS among first- and second-year medical students. *AIDS Education and Prevention*, **2**, 48–57.

22. Kyes, K. B. (1990). The effect of a 'safer sex' film as mediated by erotophobia and gender on attitudes toward condoms. *Journal of Sex Research*, **27**, 297–303.

23. Lipson, J. M. and Brown, L. T. (1991). Do videotapes improve knowledge and attitudes about AIDS? *Journal of American College Health*, **39**, 235–43.

24. Muskin, P. R. and Stevens, L. A. (1990). An AIDS educational program for third-year medical students. *General Hospital Psychiatry*, **12**, 390–5.

25. Pryor, J. B., Reeder, G. D., and McManus, J. A. (1991). Fear and loathing in the workplace: reactions to AIDS-infected co-workers. *Personality and Social Psychology Bulletin*, **17**, 133–9.

26. Rhodes, F. and Wolitski, R. (1989). Effect of instructional videotapes on AIDS knowledge and attitudes. *Journal of American College Health*, **37**, 266–71.

27. Sawyer, R. and Beck, K. H. (1991). Effects of videotapes on perceived susceptibility to HIV/AIDS among university freshmen. *Health Values*, **15**, 31–40.

Literature reviews

Healton, C. G. and Messeri, P. (1993). The effect of video interventions on improving knowledge and treatment compliance in the sexually transmitted disease clinic setting: lesson for HIV health education. *Sexually Transmitted Diseases*, **20**, 70–6.

Winett, R. A. and Anderson, E. S. (1994). HIV prevention in youth: a framework for research and action. *Advances in Clinical Child Psychology*, **16**, 1–43.

Alcohol

Adolescents

1. Bochner, S. (1994). The effectiveness of same-sex versus opposite-sex role models in advertisements to reduce alcohol consumption in teenagers. *Addictive Behaviors*, **19**, 69–82.

2. Collins, D. and Cellucci, T. (1991). Effects of a school-based alcohol education program with a media prevention component. *Psychological Reports*, **69**, 191–7.

3. Duryea, E. J. (1983). Utilizing tenets of inoculation theory to develop and evaluate a preventive alcohol education intervention. *Journal of School Health*, **53**, 250–6.

4. Duryea, E., Mohr, P., Newman, I. M., Martin, G. L., and Egwaoje, E. (1984). Six-month follow-up results of a preventive alcohol education prevention. *Journal of Drug Education*, **14**, 97–104.

5. Lignell, C. and Hizar, R. D. (1991). Effect of drug and alcohol education on attitudes of high school students. *Journal of Alcohol and Drug Education*, **37**, 31–7.

6. Alterman, A. I. and Baughman, T. G. (1991). Videotape versus computer interative education in alcoholic and nonalcoholic controls. *Alcoholism: Clinical and Experimental Research*, **15**, 39–44.

Patients

7. Baker, T. B., Udin, H., and Vogler, R. E. (1975). The effects of a videotaped modeling and self-confrontation on the drinking behavior of alcoholics. *International Journal of the Addictions*, **10**, 779–93.

8. Craigie, F. C., Jr. and Ross, S. M. (1980). The use of a videotape pretherapy training program to encourage treatment-seeking among alcohol detoxification patients. *Behavior Therapy*, **11**, 141–7.

9. Greer, R. M. and Callis, R. (1975). Use of videotape models in alcoholism rehabilitation. *Alcohol Health and Research World*, fall, 15–18.

10. McMurran, M. and Lismore, K. (1993). Using video-tapes in alcohol interventions for people with learning disabilities: an exploratory study. *Mental Handicap*, **21**, 29–31.

11. Stalonas, P. M., Keane, T. M., and Foy, D. W. (1979). Alcohol education for inpatient alcoholics: a comparison of live, videotape and written presentation modalities. *Addictive Behaviors*, **4**, 223–29.

Adults

12. Albert, W. G. and Hodgson, H. (1984). Encouraging the self-monitoring of alcohol consumption levels: the development and evaluation of 'know the score'. *Journal of Alcohol and Drug Education*, **29**, 8–18.

13. Engs, R. C. (1977). Let's look before we leap: the cognitive and behavioral evaluation of a university alcohol education program. *Journal of Alcohol and Drug Education*, **22**, 39–48.

14. McDermott, D., Tricker, R., and Farha, N. (1991). The effects of specialized training in alcohol information for counseling students. *Journal of Drug Education*, **21**, 85–94.

15. Plant, M. A., Pirie, F., and Kreitman, N. (1979). Evaluation of the Scottish health education unit's 1976 campaign on alcoholism. *Social Psychiatry*, **14**, 11–24.

16. Strickler, D. P., Bradlyn, A. S., and Maxwell, W. A. (1981). Teaching moderate drinking behaviors to young adult heavy drinkers: the effect of three training procedures. *Addictive Behaviors*, **6**, 355–64.

17. Waterson, E. J. and Murray-Lyon, I. M. (1990). Preventing fetal alcohol effects: a trial of three methods of giving information in the antenatal clinic. *Health Education Research: Theory and Practice*, **5**, 53–61.

Drugs

1. Donohew, L., Helm, D. M., Lawrence, P., and Shatzer, M. J. (1990). Sensation seeking, marijuana use and responses to prevention messages. In Watson, R. R. (ed.). *Drug and alcohol abuse prevention*. Totowa, NJ: Humana Press, pp. 73–93.

2–6. Eiser, C. and Eiser, J. R. (1988). The evaluation of 'double take': a school-based drugs education package. *Educational Review*, **40**, 349–59.

7. Hecht, M. L., Corman, S. R., and Miller-Rassulo, M. (1993) An evaluation of the 'Drug resistance project': a comparison of film versus live performance models. *Health Communication*, **5**, 75–88.

8. Vogt, A. T. (1977). Will classroom instruction change attitudes toward drug abuse? *Psychological Reports*, **41**, 973–4.

Smoking

1. Banspach, S. W., Lefebvre, R. C., and Carleton, R. A. (1989). Increasing awareness of the pressures related to smoking: an analysis of two models of anti-smoking curriculum in the classroom. *Health Education Research: Theory and Practice*, **4**, 69–78.

2. Botvin, G. J., Baker, E., Dusenbury, L., Tortu, S., and Botvin, E. M. (1990). Preventing adolescent drug abuse through a multimodal cognitive-behavioral approach: results of a 3-year study. *Journal of Consulting and Clinical Psychology*, **58**, 437–46.

3. Evans, R. I., Rozelle, R. M., Maxwell, S. E., Raines, B. E., Dill, C. A., and Guthrie, T. J. (1981). Social modeling films to deter smoking in adolescents: results of a three-year field investigation. *Journal of Applied Psychology*, **66**, 399–414.

4. Greer, R. O., Jr. (1989). Effectiveness of video instruction in educating teenagers about the health risks of smokeless tobacco use. *Journal of Cancer Education*, **4**, 33–7.

5. Hammes, M. and Petersen, D. (1986). Teaching decision-making skills to a sixth grade population. *Journal of Drug Education*, **16**, 233–41.

6. Hirschman, R. S. and Leventhal, H. (1989). Preventing smoking behavior in school children: an initial test of a cognitive-development program. *Journal of Applied Social Psychology*, **19**, 559–83.

7. Katz, R. C., Robisch, C. M., and Telch, M. J. (1989). Acquisition of smoking refusal skills in junior high school students. *Addictive Behaviors*, **14**, 201–4.

8. O'Neill, H. K., Glasgow, R. E., and McCaul, K. D. (1983). Component analysis in smoking prevention research: effects of social consequences information. *Addictive Behaviors*, **8**, 419–23

9. Patterson, C. (1984). Junior high stop smoking groups. *School Counselor*, **31**, 480–1.

10. Pfau, M., Van Bockern, S., and Kang, J. G. (1992). Use of inoculation to promote resistance to smoking initiation among adolescents. *Communication Monographs*, **59**, 213–30.

11. Pfau, M. and Van Bockern, S. (1994). The persistence of inoculation in conferring resistance to smoking initiation among adolescents. *Human Communication Research*, **20**, 413–30.

12. Schinke, S. P., Gilchrist, L. D., Schilling, R. F., Snow, W. H., and Bobo, J. K. (1986). Skills methods to prevent smoking. *Health Education Quarterly*, **13**, 23–7.

13. Sussman, S., Brannon, B. R., Flay, B. R., Gleason, L., Senor, S., Sobol, D. F., Hansen, W. B., and Johnson, C. A. (1986). The television, school and family smoking prevention/cessation project, II. Formative evaluation of television segments by teenagers and parents: implications for parental involvement in drug education. *Health Education Research: Theory and Practice*, **1**, 185–94.

14. Sussman, S., Dent, C. W., Flay, B. R., Burton, D., Craig, S., Mestel-Rauch, J., and Holden, S. (1989). Media manipulation of adolescents' personal level judgements regarding consequences of smokeless tobacco use. *Journal of Drug Education*, **19**, 43–57.

15. Telch, M. J., Miller, L. M., Killen, J. D., Cooke, S., and Maccoby, N. (1990). Social influences approach to smoking prevention: the effects of videotape delivery with and without same-age peer leader participation. *Addictive Behaviors*, **15**, 21–8.

16. Dyer, N. (1983). Smokers' luck: can a 'shocking' programme change attitudes to smoking? *Addictive Behaviors*, **8**, 43–6.

17. Hall, S. M., Bachman, J., Henderson, J. B., Barstow, R., and Jones, R. T. (1983). Smoking cessation in patients with cardiopulmonary disease: an initial study. *Addictive Behaviors*, **8**, 33–42.

18. Hallett, R. and Sutton, S. R. (1988). Intervening against smoking in the workplace. *Psychology and Health*, **2**, 13–29.

19. Lane, T. S. and Bennison, W. (1985). Reducing a resistant risk factor: analysis of an anti-smoking approach. *Patient Education and Counseling*, **7**, 367–76.

20. Lichtenstein, E. and Hollis, J. (1992). Patient referral to a smoking cessation program: who follows through? *Journal of Family Practice*, **34**, 739–44.

21. Marston, A. R. and Bettencourt, B. A. (1988). An evaluation of the American Lung Association's Home Video Cessation Program. *American Journal of Public Health*, **78**, 1226–7.

22. Pederson, L. L., Scrimgeour, W. G., and Lefcoe, N. M. (1979). Variables of hypnosis which are related to success in a smoking withdrawal program. *International Journal of Clinical and Experimental Hypnosis*, **27**, 14–20.

23. Price, J. H., Desmond, S. M., Roberts, S. M., Krol, R. A., Losh, D. P., and Snyder, F. F. (1991). Comparison of three antismoking interventions among pregnant women in an urban setting: a randomized trial. *Psychological Reports*, **68**, 595–604.

24. Reeves, B. R., Newhagen, J., Maibach, E., Basil, M., and Kurz, K. (1991). Negative and positive television messages: effects of message type and context on attention and memory. *American Behavioral Scientist*, **34**, 679–94.

25. Schwarz, N., Servay, W. and Kumpf, M. (1985). Attribution of arousal as a mediator of the effectiveness of fear-arousing communications. *Journal of Applied Social Psychology*, **15**, 178–88.

26. Stevens, V. J., Glasgow, R. E., Hollis, J. F., Lichtenstein, E., and Vogt, T. M. (1993). A smoking-cessation intervention for hospital patients. *Medical Care*, **31**, 65–72.

27. Sutton, S. R. and Eiser, J. R. (1984). The effect of fear-arousing communications on cigarette smoking: an expectancy-value approach. *Journal of Behavioral Medicine*, **7**, 13–33.

28. Watson, M., Pettingale, K. W., and Goldstein, D. (1983). Effects of a fear appeal on arousal, self-reported anxiety, and attitude towards smoking. *Psychological Reports*, **52**, 139–46.

Literature reviews

Eiser, J. R., Morgan, M., Gammage, P., Brooks, N., and Kirby, R. (1991). Adolescent health behaviour and similarity-attraction: friends share smoking habits (really), but much else besides. *British Journal of Social Psychology*, **30**, 339–48.

Flay, B. R. (1985). What we know about the social influences approach to smoking prevention: review and recommendations. *NIDA Research Monograph Series*, **63**, 67–112.

Nutrition

1. Cotugna, N. and Vickery, C. E. (1992) Development and supermarket field testing of videotaped nutrition messages for cancer risk reduction. *Public Health Reports*, **107**, 691–4.

2. Dougherty, M. F., Wittsen, A. B. and Guarino, M. A. (1990). Promoting low-fat foods in the supermarket using various methods, including videocassettes. *Journal of the American Medical Association*, **90**, 1106–8.

3. Greene, G. W. and Strychar, I. (1992). Participation in a worksite cholesterol education program in a university setting. *Journal of the American Dietetic Association*, **92**, 1376–81.

4. Lackey, C. J., Kolasa, K. M., and Horner, R. D. (1992). Nutrition education in a community cholesterol screening program. *Health Values*, **16**, 39–47.

5. Moreno, A. B. and Thelen, M. H. (1993). A preliminary prevention program for eating disorders in junior high school population. *Journal of Youth and Adolescence*, **22**, 109–24.

6. Pace, P. W., Henske, J. C., Whitfill, B. J., Andrews, S. M., Russel, M. L., Probsfield, J. L., and Insull, W., Jr. (1983). Videocassette use in diet instruction. *Journal of the American Dietetic Association*, **83**, 166–9.

7. Peterson, E. P., Jeffrey, D. B., Bridgwater, C. A., and Dawson, B. (1984). How pronutrition television programming affects children's dietary habits. *Devleopmental Psychology*, **20**, 55–63.

8. Winett, R. A., Kramer, K. D., Walker, W. B., Malone, S. W., and Lane, M. K. (1988). Modifying food purchases in supermarkets with modeling, feedback, and goal-setting procedures. *Journal of Applied Behavior Analysis*, **21**, 73–80.

9. Winett, R. A., Wagner, J. L., Moore, J. F., Walker, W. B., Hite, L. A., Leahy, M., Neubauer, T., Arbour, D., Walberg, J., Geller, E. S., Mundy, L. L., and Lombard, D. (1991a). An experimental evaluation of a prototype public access nutrition information system for supermarkets. *Health Psychology*, **10**, 75–8.

10. Winett, R. A., Moore, J. F., Wagner, J. L., Hite, L. A., Leahy, M., Neubauer, T., Walberg, J., Walker, W. B., Lombard, D., Geller, E. S., and Mundy, L. L. (1991b). Altering shoppers' supermarket purchases to fit nutritional guidelines: an interactive information system. *Journal of Applied Behavior Analysis*, **24**, 95–105.

Miscellaneous health promotion and prevention

1. Carroll-Rowan, L. A. and Miltenberger, R. G. (1994). A comparison of procedures for teaching abduction prevention to preschoolers. *Education and Treatment of Children*, **17**, 113–28.

2. Locketz, L. (1976). Health education in rural Surinam: use of videotape in a national campaign against schistosomiasis. *Bulletin of the Pan America Health Organization*, **10**, 219–26.

3. Meagher, D. and Mann, K. V. (1990). The effect of an educational program on knowledge and attitudes about blood pressure by junior high school students: a pilot project. *Canadian Journal of Cardiovascular Nursing*, **1**, 15–22.

4. Poche, C., Yoder, P. and Miltenberger, R. (1988). Teaching self-protection to children using television techniques. *Journal of Applied Behavior Analysis*, **21**, 253–61.

5. Sarason, I. G., Sarason, B. R., Pierce, G. R., Sayers, M. H., and Rosenkranz, S. L. (1992). Promotion of high school blood donations: testing the efficacy of a videotaped intervention. *Transfusion*, **32**, 818–23.

6. Sigurdson, E., Strang, M., and Doig, T. (1987). What do children know about preventing sexual assault? How can their awareness be increased? *Canadian Journal of Psychiatry*, **32**, 551–6.

7. Cody, R. and Lee, C. (1990). Behaviors, beliefs and intentions in skin cancer prevention. *Journal of Behavioural Medicine*, **13**, 373–89.

8. Hurtado, S. L. and Hovell, M. F. (1993). Efficacy of health promotion videotapes in the US navy: a lesson for health educators. *Journal of Health Education*, **24**, 107–12.

9. Miller, A. G., Ashton, W. A., McHoskey, J. W., and Gimbel, J. (1990). What price attractiveness? Stereotype and risk factors in suntanning behavior. *Journal of Applied Social Psychology*, **20**, 1272–1300.

10. Rossi, J. S., Blais, L. M., and Weinstock, M. A. (1994). The Rhode island sun smart project: skin cancer prevention reaches the beaches. *American Journal of Public Health*, **84**, 672–4.

11. Sutton, S. R. and Eiser, J. R. (1990). The decision to wear a seat belt: the role of cognitive factors, fear and prior behaviour. *Psychology and Health*, **4**, 111–23.

12. Sutton, S. and Hallett, R. (1989). Understanding seat-belt intentions and behavior: a decision-making approach. *Journal of Applied Social Psychology*, **19**, 1310–25.

Preparation for surgery

1. Bradlyn, A. S., Christoff, K., Siroka, T., O'Dell, S. T., and Harris, C. V. (1986). The effects of a videotape preparation package in reducing children's arousal and increasing cooperation during cardiac catheterization. *Behaviour Research Therapy*, **24**, 453–9.

2. Durst, L. M. (1990). Preoperative teaching videotape: the effect on children's behavior. *AORN Journal*, **52**, 576–84.

3. Elkins, P. D. and Roberts, M. C. (1985). Reducing medical fears in a general population of children: a comparison of three audiovisual modeling procedures. *Journal of Pediatric Psychology*, **10**, 65–75.

4. Melamed, B. G., Meyer, R., Gee, C., and Soule, L. (1976). The influence of time and type of preparation on children's adjustment to hospitalization. *Journal of Pediatric Psychology*, **1**, 31–7.

5. Melamed, B. G. and Siegel, L. J. (1975). Reduction of anxiety in children facing hospitalization and surgery by use of filmed modeling. *Journal of Consulting and Clinical Psychology*, **43**, 511–21.

6. Pinto, R. P. and Hollandsworth, J. G. (1989). Using videotape modeling to prepare children psychologically for surgery: influence of parents and costs versus benefits of providing preparation services. *Health Psychology*, **8**, 79–95.

7. Rasnake, L. K. and Linscheid, T. R. (1989). Anxiety reduction in children receiving medical care: developmental considerations. *Devlopmental and Behavioral Pediatrics*, **10**, 169–75.

8. Robinson, P. J. and Kobayashi, K. (1991). Development and evaluation of a presurgical preparation program. *Journal of Pediatric Psychology*, **16**, 193–212.

9. Twardosz, S., Weddle, K., Borden, L., and Stevens, E. (1986). A comparison of three methods of preparing children for surgery. *Behavior Therapy*, **17**, 14–25.

10. Uzark, K., Klos, D., Davis, W., and Rosenthal, A. (1982). Use of videotape in the preparation of children for cardiac catheterization. *Pediatric Cardiology*, **3**, 287–91.

11. Peterson, L., Schultheis, K., Ridley-Johnson, R., Miller, D. J., and Tracy, K. (1984). Comparison of three modeling procedures on the presurgical and postsurgical reactions of children. *Behavior Therapy*, **15**, 197–203.

12. Ferguson, B. F. (1979). Preparing young children for hospitalization: a comparison of two methods. *Pediatrics*, **64**, 656–64.

13. Gaskey, N. J. (1987). Evaluation of the effect of a pre-operative anesthesia videotape. *Journal of the American Association of Nurse Anesthetists*, **55**, 341–5.

14. Hawkins, R. and Price, K. (1993). The effects of an education video on patients' request for postoperative pain relief. *Australian Journal of Advanced Nursing*, **10**, 32–40.

15. Herrmann, K. S. and Kreuzer, H. (1989). A randomized prospective study on anxiety reduction by preparatory disclosure with and without video film show about a planned heart catheterization. *European Heart Journal*, **10**, 753–7.

16. Hill, N. E., Baker, M., Warner, R. A., and Taub, H. (1988). Evaluating the use of a videotape in teaching the precardiac catheterization patient. *Journal of Cardiovascular Nursing*, **2**, 71–8.

17. Holden, G., Speedling, E., and Rosenberg, G. (1992). Evaluation of an intervention designed to improve patients' hospital experience. *Psychological Reports*, **71**, 547–50.

18. Mahler, H. I. M., Kulik, J. A., and Hill, M. R. (1993). A preliminary report on the effects of videotape preparations for coronary artery bypass surgery on anxiety and self-efficacy: a simulation and validation with college students. *Basic and Applied Social Psychology*, **14**, 437–53.

19. Shipley, R. H., Butt, J. H., Horwitz, B., and Farbry, J. E. (1978). Preparation for a stressful medical procedure: effect of amount of stimulus preexposure and coping style. *Journal of Consulting and Clinical Psychology*, **46**, 499–507.

20. Wicklin, N. and Forster, J. (1994). The effects of a personal versus factual approach videotape on the level of preoperative anxiety of same day surgery patients. *Patient Education and Counseling*, **23**, 107–14.

Literature reviews

Eiser, C. (1988). Do children benefit from psychological preparation for hospitalization? *Psychology and Health*, **2**, 133–8.

Faust, J. and Melamed, B. G. (1984) Influence of arousal, experience and age on surgery preparation on same day of surgery and in-hospital pediatric patients. *Journal of Consulting and Clinical Psychology*, **52**, 359–65.

Melamed, B. G. (1977). Psychological preparation for hospitalization. In Rachman, S. *Contributions to medical psychology*, vol. 1. Elmsford, New York: Pergamon Press, pp. 47–74.

Saille, H., Burgmeier, R., and Schmidt, L. R. (1988) A meta-analysis of studies on psychological preparation of children facing medical procedures. *Psychology and Health*, **2**, 107–32.

Dentistry

1. Fields, H. and Pinkham, J. (1976). Videotape modeling of the child dental patient. *Journal of Dental Research*, **55**, 958–63.

2. Del Gaudio, D. J. and Nevid, J. S. (1991). Training dentally anxious children to cope. *Journal of Dentistry for Children*, **58**, 31–7.

3. Zachary, R. A., Friedlander, S., Huang, L. N., Silverstein, S., and Leggott, P. (1985). Effects of stress-relevant and -irrelevant filmed modeling on children's responses to dental treatment. *Journal of Pediatric Psychology*, **10**, 383–401.

4. Rouleau, J., Ladouceur, R., and Dufour, L. (1981). Pre-exposure to the first dental treatment. *Journal of Dental Research*, **60**, 30–4.

5. Klingman, A., Melamed, B. G., Cuthbert, M. I., and Hermecz, D. A. (1984). Effects of participant modeling on information acquisition and skill utilization. *Journal of Consulting and Clinical Psychology*, **52**, 414–22.

6. McMurray, N. E., Lucas, J. O., Arbes-Duprey, V., and Wright, F. A. C. (1985). The effects of mastery and coping models on stress in young children. *Australian Journal of Psychology*, **37**, 65–70.

7. Melamed, B. G., Yurcheson, R., Fleece, E. L., Hutcherson, S., and Hawes, R. (1978). Effects of film modeling on the reduction of anxiety-related behaviors in individuals varying in level of previous experience in the stress situation. *Journal of Consulting and Clinical Psychology*, **46**, 1357–67.

8. Auerbach, S. M., Kendall, P. C., Cuttler, H. F., and Levitt, N. R. (1976). Anxiety, locus of control, type of preparatory information, and adjustment to dental surgery. *Journal of Consulting and Clinical Psychology*, **44**, 809–18.

9. Davis, E. L., Albino, J. E., Tedesco, L. A., Portenoy, B. S., and Ortman, L. F. (1986). Expectations and satisfaction of denture patients in a university clinic. *Journal of Prosthetic Dentistry*, **55**, 59–63.

10. Gatchel, R. J. (1986). Impact of a videotaped dental fear-reduction program on people who avoid dental treatment. *Journal of the American Dental Association*, **112**, 218–21.

11. Kois, J., Kotch, H., Cormier, P. P., and Laster, L. (1978). The effectiveness of various methods of plaque control instruction on short-term motivation. *Journal of Preventive Dentistry*, **5**, 27–30.

12. Moore, R., Brodsgaard, I., Berggren, U., and Carlsson, S. G. (1991). Generalization of effects of dental fear treatment in a self-referred population of odontophobics. *Journal of Behavior Therapy and Experimental Psychiatry*, **22**, 243–53.

13. Robertson, C., Gatchel, R. J., and Fowler, C. (1991). Effectiveness of a videotaped behavioral intervention in reducing anxiety in emergency oral surgery patients. *Behavioral Medicine*, **17**, 77–85.

Screening

1. Banks, S. M., Salovey, P., Greener, S., Rothman, A. J., Moyer, A., Beauvais, J., and Epel, E. (1995). The effects of message framing on mammography utilization. *Health Psychology*, **14**, 178–84.

2. Ehman, J. L. (1993). BSE rap: intergenerational ties to save lives. *Oncology Nursing Forum*, **20**, 1255–9.

3. Fisher, L., Rowley P. T., and Lipkin, M. (1981). Genetic counseling for Beta-Thalassemia trait following health screening in a health maintenance organization: comparison of programmed and conventional counseling. *American Journal of Human Genetics*, **33**, 987–94.

4. Hill, D. and Gardner, G. (1980). Repression-sensitization and yielding to threatening health communications. *Australian Journal of Psychology*, **32**, 183–93.

5. McAvoy, B. R. and Raza, R. (1991). Can health education increase uptake of cervical smear testing among Asian women? *British Medical Journal*, **302**, 833–6.

6. O'Brien, S. and Lee, C. (1990). Effects of a videotape intervention on pap smear knowledge, attitudes and behaviour. *Behaviour Change*, **7**, 143–50.

7. Ser Vaas, B. and Weinberger, M. H. (1979). The use of multi-media motivation in enhancing compliance of hypertensives discovered at a screening operation. *American Journal of Public Health*, **69**, 382–4.

Patient education

Asthma

1. Holzheimer, L., Mohay, H., and Masters, B. (1995). A comparison of written versus video taped materials for teaching young children about asthma management. *Proceedings of the Seventh National Health Promotion Conference*, Queensland State Education Department, Brisbane, Queensland, February 1995.

2. Moldofsky, H., Broder, I., Davies, G., and Leznoff, A. (1979). Videotape educational program for people with asthma. *Canadian Medical Association Journal*, **120**, 669–72.

3. Partridge, M. R. (1986). Asthma education: more reading or more viewing? *Journal of the Royal Society of Medicine*, **79**, 326–8.

Renal disease

4. Barbour, G. L. and Blumenkrantz, M. J. (1978). Videotape aids informed consent decision. *Journal of the American Medical Association*, **240**, 2741–2.

5. Lawson, V. K., Taylor, M. N. and Gram, M. R. (1976). An audio-tutorial aid for dietary instruction in renal dialysis. *Journal of the American Dietetic Association*, **69**, 390–6.

Diabetes

6. Bethea, C. D., Stallings, S. F., Wolman, P. G., and Ingram, R. C. (1989). Comparison of conventional and videotaped diabetic exchange lists instruction. *Journal of the American Dietetic Association*, **89**, 405–6.

7. Brown, S. A., Duchin, S. P., and Villagomez, E. T. (1992). Diabetes education in a Mexican-American population: pilot testing of a research-based videotape. *Diabetes Educator*, **18**, 47–51.

8. Gilbert, B. O., Johnson, S. B., Spillar, R., McCallum, M., Silverstein, J. H., and Rosenbloom, A. (1982). The effects of a peer-modeling film on children learning to self-inject insulin. *Behavior Therapy*, **13**, 186–93.

9. McCulloch, D. K., Mitchell, R. D., Ambler, J., and Tattersall, R. B. (1983). Influence of imaginative teaching of diet on compliance and metabolic control in insulin dependent diabetes. *British Medical Journal*, **287**, 1858–61.

10. McCulloch, D. K., Mitchell, R. D., Ambler, J., and Tattersall, R. B. (1985). A prospective comparison of 'conventional' and high carbohydrate/high fibre/low fat diets in adults with established type 1 (insulin dependent) diabetes. *Diabetologia*, **28**, 208–12.

11. Pichert, J. W., Snyder, G. M., Kinzer, C. K., and Boswell, E. J. (1994). Problem solving anchored instruction about sick days for adolescents with diabetes. *Patient Education and Counseling*, **23**, 115–24.

Cardiac conditions

12. Bracken, M. B., Bracken, M, and Landry, A. B. (1977). Patient education by videotape after myocardial infarction: an empirical evaluation. *Archives of Physical Medicine and Rehabilitation*, **58**, 213–19.

13. Brandao, J. J., Brademan, G. M., Moore, C. E., Wright, D., and Kleiman, N. S. (1992). Effectiveness of videotaped dietary instruction for patients hospitalized with cardiovascular disease. *Journal of the American Dietetic Association*, **92**, 1268–70.

Miscellaneous

14. Anderson, L. A., DeVellis, B. M., and DeVellis, R. F. (1987). Effects of modeling on patient communication, satisfaction and knowledge. *Medical Care*, **25**, 1044–56.

15. Barry, S. P. and Daniels, A. A. (1984) Effecting change in outpatient failed appointments. *Journal of Family Practice*, **18**, 739–42.

16. Buckley, K., Plaut, S. M., and Ruley, E. J. (1981). Teaching home monitoring of blood pressure to adolescents. *Adolescence*, **16**, 881–9.

17. Hamilton, G. A., Roberts, S. J., Johnson, J. M., Tropp, J. R., Anthony-Odgren, D., and Johnson, B. F. (1993). Increasing adherence in patients with primary hypertension: an intervention. *Health Values*, **17**, 3–11.

18. Koperski, M. (1989). Health education using video recordings in a general practice waiting area: an evaluation. *Journal of the Royal College of General Practitioners*, **39**, 328–30.

19. McGowan, M. P., Joffe, A., Duggan, A. K., and McCay, P. S. (1994). Intervention in hypercholesterolemic college students: a pilot study. *Journal of Adolescent Health*, **15**, 155–62.

20. Rosenthal, A. R., Zimmerman, J. F., and Tanner, J. (1983). Educating the glaucoma patient. *British Journal of Ophthalmology*, **67**, 814–17.

21. Sanguinetti, M. and Catanzaro, M. (1987). A comparison of discharge teaching on the consequences of brain injury. *Journal of Neuroscience Nursing*, **19**, 271–5.

22. Stone, S., Holden, A., Knapic, N., and Ansell, J. (1989). Comparison between videotape and personalized patient education for anticoagulant therapy. *Journal of Family Practice*, **29**, 55–7.

Literature reviews

Bradley, C. (ed.) (1994). *Handbook of psychology and diabetes: a guide to psychological measurement in diabetes research and practice*. Reading, Berks.: Harwood Academic Publishers.

Parenting

Pregnancy and labour

1. Bachman, J. W., Field, C. S., and Hammersley, C. E. (1992). Educational program for premature labor. *Journal of the American Board of Family Practice*, **5**, 645–7.

2. Cobiella, C. W., Mabe, P. A., and Forehand, R. L. (1990). A comparison of two-stress reduction treatments for mothers of neonates hospitalized in a neonatal intensive care unit. *Children's Health Care*, **19**, 93–100.

3. Daelhousen, B. B and Guthrie, H. A. (1982). A self-instruction nutrition program for pregnant women. *Journal of the American Dietetic Association*, **81**, 407–12.

4. Freda, M. C., Damus, K., Andersen, H. F., Brustman, L. E., and Merkatz, I. R. (1990). A 'PROPP' for the Bronx: preterm birth prevention education in the inner city. *Obstetrics & Gynecology*, **76**, 935–56.

5. Freda, M. C., Damus, K., and Merkatz, I. R. (1988). The urban community as the client in preterm birth prevention: evaluation of a program component. *Social Sciences and Medicine*, **27**, 1439–46.

6. Manderino, M. A. and Bzdek, V. M. (1984). Effects of modelling and information on reactions to pain: a childbirth-preparation analogue. *Nursing Research*, **33**, 9–14.

7. Mynaugh, P. A. (1991). A randomized study of two methods of teaching perineal massage: effects on practice rates, episiotomy rates, and lacerations. *Birth*, **18**, 153–9.

Parent education

8. Kleemeier, C. P. and Hazzard, A. P. (1984). Videotaped parent education in pediatric waiting rooms. *Patient Education and Counseling*, **6**, 122–4.

9. Koniak-Griffin, D., Verzemnieks, I., and Cahill, D. (1992). Using videotape instruction and feedback to improve adolescents' mothering behaviors. *Journal of Adolescent Health*, **13**, 570–5.

10. Paperny, D. (1992). Pediatric medical advice enhanced with use of video. *AJDC: American Journal of Diseases of Children*, **146**, 785–6.

11. Rossiter, J. C. (1994). The effect of a culture-specific education program to promote breastfeeding among Vietnamese women in Sydney. *International Journal of Nursing Studies*, **31**, 369–79.

General references

Ajzen, I. (1991). The theory of planned behavior. *Organizational Behavior and Decision Processes*, **50**, 1–33.

Ajzen, I. and Fishbein, M. (1980) *Understanding attitudes and predicting social behavior*. Englewood Cliffs, NJ: Prentice-Hall.

Bandura, A. (1971). *Social learning theory*. Morristown, NJ: General Learning Press.

Bandura, A. (1977). Self-efficacy: toward a unifying theory of behavioral change. *Psychological Review*, **84**, 1919–2015.

Bandura, A. (1986). *Social foundations of thought and action: a social cognitive theory*. Englewood Cliffs, NJ: Prentice-Hall.

Becker, M. H. (ed.) (1974). The health belief model and personal health behavior. *Health Education Monographs*, **2**, 324–473.

Bradley, C. (ed.) (1994). *Handbook of psychology and diabetes: a guide to psychological measurement in diabetes research and practice*. Reading, Berks.: Harwood Academic Publishers.

Clabots, R. B. and Dolphin, D. (1992). The Multilingual Videotape Project: community involvement in a unique health education program. *Public Health Reports*, **107**, 75–80.

Cohen, S. A. (1981). Patient education: a review of the literature. *Journal of Advanced Nursing*, **6**, 11–8.

Corah, N. L.(1969). Development of a dental anxiety scale. *Journal of Dental Research*, **48**, 596.

Curry, R. L. and Cullen, J. C. (1990). Using videorecordings in pediatric nursing practice. *Pediatric Nursing*, **16**, 501–4.

Deane, F. P., Spicer, J., and Leatham, J. (1992). Effects of videotaped preparatory information on expectations, anxiety and psychotherapy outcome. *Journal of Consulting and Clinical Psychology*, **60**, 980–4.

Donaldson, S. I., Graham, J. W., Piccinin, A. M., and Hansen, W. B. (1995). Resistance-skills training and onset of alcohol use: evidence for beneficial and potentially harmful effects in public schools and in private catholic schools. *Health Psychology*, **14**, 291–300.

Dowrick, P. W. and Raeburn, J. M.(1976). Video editing and medication to produce a therapeutic self model – case study. *Journal of Consulting and Clinical Psychology*, **45**, 1156–8.

Dowrick, P. W. (1991). *Practical guide to using video in the behavioural sciences*. New York: Wiley.

Eiser, J. R., Morgan, M., Gammage, P., Brooks, N., and Kirby, R.(1991). Adolescent health behaviour and similarity-attraction: friends share smoking habits (really), but much else besides. *British Journal of Social Psychology*, **30**, 339–48.

Forth Valley Health Board, Department of Community Medicine and Nursing Services, Scottish Health Education Group (1991). *Health learning through video: the Scottish experience with patients/clients*. Stirling: Forth Valley Health Board.

Gagliano, M. E. (1988). A literature review on the efficacy of video in patient education. *Journal of Medical Education*, **63**, 785–92.